Self Assessment
Questions and Answers
for Dental Assistants

Second Edition

Self Assessment Questions and Answers for Dental Assistants

Second Edition

Peter L. Erridge, LDS, RCS(Eng.)
Dental Surgeon
Guy's Hospital, St Thomas Street, London
Panel Member, UK Examining Board
for Dental Surgery Assistants

Wright

Wright
An imprint of Butterworth-Heinemann Ltd
Linacre House, Jordan Hill, Oxford OX2 8DP

 PART OF REED INTERNATIONAL BOOKS

OXFORD   LONDON   BOSTON
MUNICH   NEW DELHI   SINGAPORE   SYDNEY
TOKYO   TORONTO   WELLINGTON

First published 1979
Second edition 1988
Reprinted 1992 (twice) , 1993

© Butterworth-Heinemann Ltd 1988

British Library Cataloguing in Publication Data
Erridge, P. (Peter L.)
    Self assessment questions and answers
    for dental assistants — 2nd ed.
    1. Dentistry — Questions and answers — For
    dental assistants
    I. Title
    617.6'0076

ISBN 0 7236 0963 2

Library of Congress Cataloguing in Publication Data
Erridge, Peter L.
    Self assessment questions and answers for dental assistants/
    P. L. Erridge. — 2nd ed.
    p. cm.
    ISBN 0 7236 0963 2
    1. Dental assistants — Examinations, questions, etc.
    2. Dentistry — Examinations, questions, etc. I. Title
    [DNLM: 1. Dental Assistants — examination questions.
    WU 18.5 E72s]
    RK60.5.E77   1988
    DNLM/DLC
    for Library of Congress   88-10606

Printed and bound in Great Britain by
Antony Rowe Limited, Chippenham, Wiltshire

Preface to the second edition

The opportunity has been taken to meet some of the criticisms of the earlier edition, to add questions on new techniques and materials and to take account of the change of emphasis in dental care. The Report of the Dental Surgery Assistants Standards and Training Advisory Board of the United Kingdom has been used as a guide to the scope of the questions.

It is hoped that users will find the new layout to be an improvement whilst resisting the temptation to refer too quickly to the answers. Again the author wishes to emphasize the importance of writing down the answers before checking since it is so easy to decide that the 'thought answer' corresponds to the answer in the book.

I wish to thank my colleagues who kindly read the manuscript and gave many helpful suggestions, the dental assistants who took part in testing the multiple choice questions and my wife for her advice and continued forbearance during the preparation of this second edition.

Preface to the first edition

There are two stages in the learning process: firstly, learning the facts, secondly, trying to understand these facts and applying them to everyday work. Experience in teaching and in examining dental assistants has shown that much time is spent trying to assimilate the facts but not enough effort is expended on their understanding and application.

Therefore it was considered that a book was needed which would encourage the dental assistants to question basic facts with the basic questions: how, what, where, when and why. Furthermore, it is hoped that having been encouraged to have a questioning attitude, the students will maintain and develop this approach to work to the advantage of themselves and to the practice of dentistry.

Some difficulty is always experienced in deciding the level of knowledge and understanding which a dental assistant should acquire. The author hopes that an acceptable compromise has been reached and would be pleased to receive comments from students and teachers.

How to use this book

It is suggested that the student reads the relevant section in the textbooks, attends the lecture (if possible) and then reads the textbook again. Only after learning as much as possible about that particular subject should any attempt be made to answer questions in this book, if maximum benefit is to be gained. It is recommended that all the questions on one subject are answered before reference is made to the answer section.

The major part of the book consists of basic questions requiring concise answers. For accuracy of self-marking it is recommended that answers to each question be written down. In this way differences between what was intended and what was actually expressed will be noted and this should benefit the learning process.

There is a short section on instrument and material layouts for practical procedures. It is important that the lists are written in the order of use as this helps to show understanding of the procedures and to obviate omissions.

Another part is entitled 'Short Essay Questions'. Each question should be answered with a short essay giving relevant facts in concise sentences. Only when the written answer is as good as it can be should reference be made to the model answers. The model answers contain a skeleton answer together with a marking scheme. The marks give some indication of the relative importance of the facts to the answer.

The answers to these sections have been kept as concise as possible which will in some cases lead the student to need further information. Reference back to the standard textbooks will clarify most issues. In all cases it is to be hoped that the student will be given maximum support and encouragement by the dental surgeon.

The final part contains multiple choice questions. In these questions a statement is made or a question is asked. Underneath, several possible answers are given, *one or more* of which can be considered the most appropriate answer. This type of question depends upon accuracy of meaning of words both in the question and in the answer. Great care has beeen taken in devising the questions but it may be that some students will experience problems–the author hopes these will be few. Note should be made of the answers to a complete section before referring to the answers. This section could be used as final revision.

Contents

General, including duties

Questions

1. Accuracy is very important with patient records–why is this?
2. After a general dental examination, what special examinations might be required for a patient?
3. What should the dental assistant (DA) check at re-examination appointments?
4. Why are patients asked if they have had jaundice or hepatitis?
5. Why does the dental surgeon wish to know if the patient is pregnant?
6. Name the official body responsible for the licensing, regulation and control of the practice of dentistry in the UK.
7. Who is allowed by law to carry out dental procedures within the mouth?
8. Under what circumstances can the DA give oral hygiene advice to a patient?
9. When can the DA take radiographs?

Answers

1. (a) Medical notes–inaccurate or incomplete records can put lives at risk
   (b) The right patient must receive the right treatment on the right tooth
   (c) Information on past treatment can assist current treatment
   (d) Claims for fees are based on the records
   (e) It could be important medico-legally

2. (a) Dental radiographs
   (b) Use of disclosing dyes
   (c) Vitality tests
   (d) Assessment and charting for the periodontal or orthodontic condition
   (e) Biopsy of tissue
   (f) Medical tests e.g. pulse, temperature, blood pressure, haematology etc.

3. (a) That correct notes are out for the patient who has attended
   (b) If there has been any change in the details, address, telephone etc.

4. Jaundice is a yellow coloration of the skin due to a variety of causes one of which is liver disease or hepatitis. There are several causes of hepatitis one of which is hepatitis B virus, but about half those people contracting hepatitis B do not show signs of the condition. For this reason precautions should be taken with all patients.

5. (a) Protection–to avoid the risk of exposure to radiation
           –care in prescribing or administration of drugs which might affect the foetus
   (b) Treatment–simplification of treatment plan e.g. put off long or difficult procedures
   (c) Advice   –on care of mouth during pregnancy
                –reinforce dental prevention advice

6. The General Dental Council

7. Registered dental surgeons. Registered therapists and hygienists can carry out certain procedures prescribed by the dental surgeon

8. If he/she has been instructed by the dental surgeon in the methods and materials suitable to the patient

9. Under EEC regulations, radiographs should be taken only by a person who has received training and passed a suitable examination in radiography

10. What active role can the DA take in the administration of a general anaesthetic?

11. What should the DA check at the end of a general anaesthetic before the patient starts to recover?

12. What is the legal position of a DA giving assistance in an emergency situation?

13. What is the legal role of the DA in the handling of drugs?

14. If a patient asks for a copy of his/her dental notes—what should the DA do?

15. What is the legal role of the DA in the surgery?

16. In the event of a DA being present when there is a dentist–patient problem, what should the DA do?

17. What should the Receptionist check when a patient arrives at the surgery?

10. Only as an assistant to the anaesthetist in ways such as helping the patient or passing and holding equipment

11. That all instruments, cotton wool rolls, swabs and extracted teeth are accounted for

12. That of a member of the general public with training as a first aider–to call for professional assistance then to give first aid

13. Apart from simple 'home' type drugs, none. Any other duties in this area must be under the direct personal supervision of a dentist or doctor

14. Pass the request to the dental surgeon, who is the only person who should authorize copies

15. As a chaperone and as a witness

16. Remain in the surgery and try to memorize events and words. It could be useful to make some personal notes of the episode

17. (a) That he/she has an appointment
    (b) That it is correct for day and time
    (c) That the patient has followed any instructions e.g. bringing money or toothbrush, nil by mouth etc.
    (d) Whether the operator is running late and if so, to advise the patient
    (e) That the patient knows where to find the waiting room and toilet and the 'house rules' regarding smoking, leaving personal property e.g. coats

18. List, in a logical order, the duties of the DA for each of the following:

A. At the start and end of each working day
B. In regard to petty cash

18A Start of day
   General duties
   (a) On arrival, visually check exterior for signs of damage before opening the door
   (b) Switch off the alarm and the isolating main switch
   (c) Check the internal security, switch on main services, attend to the heating and ventilation
   (d) Switch on major equipment e.g. compressor, sterilizer, dental unit
   (e) Check cleaning carried out, if not then it will need to be done
   Surgery duties
   (a) Wash hands, damp dust all surfaces and equipment followed by antiseptic wipe for equipment and working surfaces
   (b) Test all equipment by running it, report any problems
   (c) Check record cards against day list, locate any which are missing
   (d) Wash hands, prepare trays for the first few patients
   (e) Lay out materials and supplies and have laboratory work ready
   (f) Lay out clean coat for the operator
   End of day
   Surgery duties
   (a) Clean instruments from the last patient and items which are sterilizable e.g. 3-in-1 syringe nozzle, handpieces and place them in the sterilizer and start the cycle
   (b) Clean and oil handpieces–if suitable they should be included in the sterilizer load; if not, then antiseptic cleaning
   (c) Wash hands, put away all materials and supplies etc.
   (d) Clean and wash down with antiseptic all equipment and working surfaces
   (e) Flush spittoon and suction with non-foaming antiseptic and leave antiseptic in the system overnight
   (f) Empty wastebin and place new liner, wash hands
   (g) Pack up all laboratory work; check laboratory work required for the next day is ready
   (h) Empty sterilizer and place items in storage
   (i) Switch off all services and make the surgery secure

18B (a) To record all transactions, income as well as expenditure
   (b) To produce a daily balance and report any discrepancies
   (c) To ensure the security of the cash during the day and overnight

19. List, in a logical order, the duties of the DA for each of the following:
  A. For security and safety at the end of the day
  B. At an examination appointment
  C. For close support dentistry
  D. To assist in the taking of dental X-ray films

19A(a) Surgery: (i) lock away drugs and prescription pads; (ii) switch off electrical apparatus; (iii) secure all windows
(b) Office: (i) observe overnight cash security arrangements; (ii) switch off electrical apparatus; (iii) close all filing cabinets securely; (iv) secure all windows
(c) Building: (i) doors and windows–check that all are securely locked; (ii) electrical–operate isolating main switch, if one is installed; (iii) exterior–check all windows closed and gates locked; (iv) alarm system–if present, set and leave premises locking the exit door securely

19B(a) Wash hands at start and as necessary
(b) Prepare the surgery by laying out instruments and materials
(c) Have available the record card and any radiographs
(d) Show the patient to the chair, leaving personal items in the appropriate place and have the patient ready for the operator
(e) Assist in recording notes as dictated by the operator
(f) Assist in the examination as required e.g by passing instruments, by retraction of tissues, cleaning and drying teeth using the 3-in-1 syringe
(g) Assist at any special tests or examinations e.g. radiography
(h) Arrange any further appointments
(i) Clear and clean the surgery before preparing for the next patient

19C(a) As far as possible, prepare in advance for the procedure
(b) Passing and exchange of instruments
(c) Retraction and protection of soft tissues
(d) Irrigation and aspiration of mouth fluids and debris to maintain a clean operating site
(e) Maintaining a clear view for the operator, including adjustment of the operating light
(f) Mixing and passing of materials
(g) Monitoring the patient
(h) By anticipation try to ensure a smooth efficient procedure

19D(a) Prepare the X-ray machine–position close to the chair, switch on, set the timer
(b) Prepare the film and if needed a holder
(c) Prepare the patient–adjust position of chair and neck rest–place the lead apron on the patient
(d) Ensure that other persons leave the room
(e) Stand at least 2 metres to the side or behind the machine during exposure
(f) After exposure–switch off the machine, move it to the store position
(g) Remove lead apron
(h) Dry films, write patient's name on them and store ready for processing at the earliest opportunity

Oral Anatomy

Questions

1. Which bones form the major part of the upper jaw?
2. Which bony cavity is part of the upper jaw?
3. Which part of the upper jaw forms the floor of the nose?
4. Occasionally the roof of the mouth does not develop properly in a baby. What is this abnormality called?
5. The roots of which teeth sometimes form part of the floor of the antrum?
6. What is a foramen?
7. What is the alveolar bone?
8. What is the alveolar ridge?
9. After a dental clearance the jawbone shrinks—what is this process called?
10. Where is the soft palate found?
11. What are the functions of the soft palate?
12. Name the ridges of tissue in the roof of the mouth. What is their function?
13 What is the name applied to the soft tissue lining the oral cavity?
14. The ascending ramus of the mandible has two prominent parts. What are they called and what is their function?
15. Give the name of the opening on the inner surface of the mandible. What is its function?
16. What is meant by the following terms:
    (a) periosteum?
    (b) maxillary tuberosity?
    (c) buccal sulcus?
17. Where can the DA feel his/her own temporo-mandibular joint?
18. How can a dislocated (subluxated) jaw be recognized?

Answers

1. Left and right maxilla
2. The maxillary antrum
3. The palate
4. Cleft palate
5. The upper posteriors, usually the first permanent molars
6. A natural opening on the surface of a bone
7. The spongy tooth-bearing bone of both jaws
8. The compact bone which remains after the extraction of teeth and the healing of the sockets
9. Resorption
10. At the posterior edge of the hard palate
11. (a) To close the nasal cavity from the mouth, so preventing food and liquids getting into the nose
    (b) It aids speech
12. Rugae. They assist in formation of speech
13. Mucous membrane
14. (a) Coronoid process–attachment of the temporal muscle
    (b) Condyle–articulation with the base of the skull. It forms part of the temporo-mandibular joint
15. Mandibular foramen. It allows the passage of the inferior dental nerve and blood vessels
16. (a) The fibrous tissue immediately covering the bone; it is essential to the nutrition of bone
    (b) The rounded posterior end of the maxillary alveolar bone
    (c) The gutter of mucous membrane between the alveolus and the cheek
17. Place a finger on the skin about 1 cm in front of the external auditory orifice. When the mouth is slightly opened and closed the movement of the condyle in the joint can be felt
18. The mouth is open and cannot be closed. The mandible is protruded

19. What is the first aid treatment of a subluxated mandible?

20. Where is the mental foramen to be found in the dentate adult?

21. After giving a mandibular nerve local anaesthetic block the operator may ask the patient if their lip is numb–why is this question asked?

22. What are the functions of the mucous membrane?

23. What are the main functions of the tongue?

24. Where are the salivary glands situated?

25. What are the main functions of saliva?

26. What causes the increase and decrease in the flow of saliva?

27. Swelling of the parotid gland is usually associated with which condition?

28. Name the muscles mainly concerned with closure of the jaws?

29. Which muscle is mainly concerned with helping to swing the mandible to either side?

30. Which muscles control lip movements?

31. Why is the mylohyoid muscle important in denture construction?

32. The muscles of mastication are supplied by which nerve?

33. Which cranial nerve supplies the teeth and jaws, and what are its three main branches?

34. Sensory nerves of the lower lip are part of which nerve?

35. Why does the tongue usually go numb after an inferior dental nerve block has been given?

19. (a) Try to get the person to relax to allow the jaw to slip naturally back into position
   (b) If this is not successful seek professional help
   (c) Following correction the person is advised to avoid opening the mouth more than a centimetre during the next few hours to prevent recurrence

20. On the outer surface of the mandible between the apices of the premolar teeth

21. Numbness indicates that the mental nerve has been anaesthetized and this nerve is an end-branch of the inferior dental nerve which supplies the mandibular teeth

22. (a) As a barrier against micro-organisms
   (b) To produce mucus for protection against mechanical injury of the oropharynx
   (c) Sensory nerve endings e.g. touch and taste, for protection

23. (a) To assist in mastication and swallowing
   (b) As an organ of sensation
   (c) In speech

24. (a) Parotid–in front of the ear
   (b) Submandibular–inside (lingual to) the angle of the mandible
   (c) Sublingual–under the anterior part of the floor of the mouth

25. Protection, lubrication, cleansing, aid to speech, digestion of starch

26. Increase can be due to the sight or smell of food, teething, or objects in the mouth
   Decrease can be due to disease, nervousness, or some drugs

27. Mumps

28. The temporal, masseter and medial pterygoid muscles

29. The lateral pterygoid

30. Muscles of facial expression

31. It forms the floor of the mouth and can cause a lower denture to lift off the alveolar ridge

32. Motor fibres of the mandibular division of the trigeminal nerve

33. Fifth (V) or trigeminal. Ophthalmic, maxillary, mandibular

34. Mental branch of the inferior dental nerve–a branch of cranial V

35. The lingual nerve, a branch of the mandibular nerve, passes close to the inferior dental foramen. The anaesthetic solution deposited in that area will usually affect the lingual nerve

36. To extract a permanent lower second molar tooth under local anaesthesia, the operator will give the patient which injections and why?

37. How does the density of the bone in the area of the mandibular permanent molars affect the local anaesthesia technique used by dental surgeons?

38. Name the branches to the palate of the maxillary nerve

39. When the jaw moves from open to closed, what muscle actions take place?

36. (a) Mandibular nerve block, to anaesthetize the tooth and lingual gum

   (b) Infiltration buccal to the teeth also will be needed, to anaesthetize the long buccal nerve which is the sensory nerve to the buccal gum

37. This bone is very dense and an infiltration anaesthetic produces little analgesia of the teeth: therefore a regional anaesthetic is given.

38. Naso-palatine, greater and lesser palatine nerves

39. The infra-mandibular muscles relax and the muscles of mastication contract.

Tooth anatomy

Questions

1. Which surface of a tooth touches the following:
   (a) the lips?
   (b) the cheek?
   (c) the tooth in front?
   (d) the gingivae?
   (e) the lower surface of the side of the tongue?
   (f) the upper surface of the side of the tongue?
   (g) the tooth behind?
   (h) the opposing teeth?

2. At what age do (a) deciduous and (b) permanent teeth start to form?

3. What is a tooth germ?

4. Which substances help in the formation of teeth?

5. Visually, how do deciduous teeth differ from permanent teeth?

6. At what age do the deciduous teeth normally start to erupt?

7. By what age should the first dental examination take place. Why this age?

8. Why do deciduous teeth have divergent roots?

9. Which type of teeth have no deciduous predecessors?

10. Define the following words:
    (a) exfoliation
    (b) dentate
    (c) edentate

11. Which tissues constitute the crown of a tooth?

12. Which tissues constitute the root of a tooth?

13. How is a tooth held in its socket?

14. What is the apical foramen and where is it usually found?

15. Where is the inter-radicular bone found?

16. In tooth anatomy, what is the bifurcation?

17. Which dental tissue lines the walls of pits and fissures?

18. Ameloblasts form which type of tissue?

19. Where is enamel thicker?

Answers

1. (a) Labial
   (b) Buccal
   (c) Mesial
   (d) Cervical
   (e) Lingual
   (f) Palatal
   (g) Distal
   (h) Occlusal

2. (a) About the sixth week after conception
   (b) About the 18th week after conception

3. A group of tissues from which a tooth develops

4. Calcium, phosphates, vitamin A and D

5. Deciduous teeth
   (a) are smaller and white
   (b) have more bulbous crowns
   (c) have divergent roots
   (d) have proportionally a larger pulp chamber

6. Six months after birth

7. Three years. Normally all the deciduous teeth will have erupted

8. To allow space for the permanent successors to develop

9. Premolars

10. (a) Natural loss of the deciduous teeth
    (b) Having some or all of the natural teeth present
    (c) Without any natural teeth

11. Enamel, dentine and pulp

12. Cementum, dentine and pulp

13. By the periodontal ligament which is attached to the cementum and to the bone forming the socket wall

14. The opening through which blood vessels and nerves enter the tooth at or near the apex of each root of each tooth

15. Between the roots of the teeth

16. Where the roots of the teeth divide

17. Enamel

18. Enamel

19. On occlusal surfaces and at cusps

20. What is meant by enamel hypoplasia?

21. Give the main causes of enamel hypoplasia.

22. What is an odontoblast?

23. Why can enamel not be formed after eruption of the tooth?

24. What is the name given to the area where the enamel and dentine join?

25. Briefly, what is the microscopic structure of enamel?

26. How is pain conducted to the pulp?

27. Which dental tissue contains millions of fibres, and what is their function?

28. How does the size of the pulp of a permanent tooth alter during life?

29. The tooth pulp contains several types of tissue–give their names.

30. Which permanent teeth commonly have:
   (a) no cusps?
   (b) one cusp?
   (c) four cusps?
   (d) five cusps?
   (e) a cusp of Carabelli?
   (f) a conical root?
   (g) a flattened root?
   (h) two roots?
   (i) three roots?
   (j) four roots?

31. What is a dental contact point?

32. Name the area between the contact points and the alveolar bone.

33. What dental structure normally fills this space?

34. Why is this area important?

35. Which are usually the first permanent teeth to erupt and at about what age?

36. What is the clinical crown of a tooth?

37. What is the normal number of (a) deciduous (b) permanent teeth

20. Defective enamel due to interference with the enamel formation process

21. Infection–local e.g. abscess of deciduous predecessor
    –general e.g. serious illness when teeth were being formed
    Trauma –injury to deciduous tooth affecting the developing successor

22. A dentine forming cell

23. The ameloblasts lie on the outer surface of the enamel and are destroyed when the tooth erupts

24. Amelo–dentinal junction

25. Rods or prisms radiating from the dentine and composed of calcium salts

26. Via dentinal tubules along the odontoblastic process

27. The periodontal ligament. To hold the tooth in position in its socket

28. Secondary dentine can be laid down, reducing the size of the pulp chamber

29. Nerves, blood vessels and connective tissue

30. (a) Incisors
    (b) Canines
    (c) Second molars
    (d) First molars
    (e) Upper first permanent molars
    (f) Upper canines and central incisors
    (g) Lower incisors
    (h) Lower molars and upper first premolars
    (i) Upper molars
    (j) Sometimes lower first permanent molars

31. The area where two adjacent teeth touch. Usually only enamel is involved

32. The interdental area

33. The interdental papilla

34. It is a stagnation area in which caries and periodontal disease can start

35. Lower central incisors or first molars. About six years

36. The part of the tooth visible in the mouth

37. (a) 20 (b) 32

38. Give the principles of the European and International (FDI) systems of charting the permanent dentition

39. How are the deciduous teeth notated on a charting?

40. What is the name given to extra teeth?

41. What is meant by the expressions (a) DMF and (b) DMFS?

38. (a) European–numbers 1 to 8 placed in a quadrant grid --/--. Numbering starts at the mid-line in each quadrant

(b) FDI–each quadrant is given a prefix number, thus: upper right = 1; upper left = 2; lower right = 4; lower left = 3 Each tooth is given the same number as in the European system.

39. Usually by an alphabetic system

40. Supernumerary teeth–usually charted 'S' between the normal teeth

41. (a) decayed, missing or filled teeth

(b) FDI–each quadrant is given a prefix number, thus: upper right = 1; upper left = 2;lower right = 4, lower left = 3 Each tooth is given the same number as in the European system.

Microbiology and pathology

Questions

1. Define the following words:
   (a) microbiology
   (b) non-pathogenic
   (c) bacteriostasis
   (d) spore

2. Name three main groups of non-pathogenic micro-organisms and give examples of their uses

3. What is the approximate size of (a) bacteria and (b) viruses?

4. How may infection be spread?

5. What are the ideal living conditions for most micro-organisms?

6. What are anaerobic micro-organisms?

7. Where, about the body, are micro-organisms most commonly found?

8. How may micro-organisms enter the body?

9. What is meant by a 'carrier' of infection?

10. What factors increase the chances of a person developing an infection?

11. How do micro-organisms cause disease?

Answers

1. (a) Study of living organisms which are visible to the human eye only through a microscope
   (b) Not causing disease
   (c) When numbers of bacteria remain constant
   (d) A protective state for micro-organisms to withstand unfavourable conditions

2. (a) Saprophytes–aid decomposition
   (b) Bacteria–aid digestion
   (c) Fungi–yeasts–ferment e.g. wine and bread
         moulds–produce antibiotics

3. (a) One-thousandth of a millimetre
   (b) One-millionth of a millimetre

4. (a) Inoculation of body surfaces
      (i) Direct contact e.g. person to person
      (ii) Indirect contact–through an intermediate agent such as a mouthwash glass or via animals e.g. biting insects
   (b) Inhalation into respiratory tract
      (i) Droplet infection
      (ii) Dust particles
   (c) Ingestion into digestive tract: solids, liquids

5. Nutrients, moisture, lack of sunlight, correct temperature and correct level of oxygen

6. Those which need little or no oxygen for normal living conditions

7. Skin folds, under nails, on hair, in body openings and tracts

8. Through body surfaces e.g. respiratory or alimentary tracts, damaged skin or mucous membrane

9. A person who carries the micro-organism which causes a particular disease but does not show signs of the disease.

10. (a) Virulence of micro-organisms
    (b) A massive number of pathogens
    (c) Resistance of individual
       (i) General factors e.g. health, age
       (ii) Passive–surface defences e.g. skin, mucous membranes
       (iii) Active–tissue defences–serous exudate dilutes and carries away infection and brings both antibodies and white cells

11. (a) They invade and multiply within the body using nutrients and oxygen meant for body cells
    (b) They may obstruct blood vessels and ducts
    (c) Their waste products may be harmful to the body tissues.

12. What is the result of most everyday infections of humans?

13. How can the DA help to cause disease in the mouth?

14. What is the name of the condition in which micro-organisms are present in the bloodstream without clinical symptoms?

15. Most mouths contain pathologic organisms but few have serious soft tissue disease–why is this?

16. What is meant by immunity?

17. What is the cause of lockjaw?

18. What is a virus?

19. How do viruses affect a living body?

20. Give the names of at least two conditions caused by viruses which are of interest to dentists

21. What is meant by 'cross-infection'?

22. In general, which groups of people are considered to include individuals with a high risk of infection?

23. Which organisms are associated with the following:
    (a) enamel caries?
    (b) dentine caries?
    (c) acute ulcerative gingivitis?
    (d) denture sore mouth?

24. What is pus and what does it contain?

25. What is a collection of pus called?

26. In dentistry particular care is taken against spreading which blood-borne liver disease?

12. No discomfort or clinical symptoms because the number of micro-organisms is below the threshold necessary for disease to occur.

13. (a) Inadequate sterilization leading to cross-infection
    (b) Accidental use of unsterile instruments or materials e.g. partly used anaesthetic cartridge

14. Bacteraemia

15. Provided that there is no break in the mucosa the body is able to deal with most infections. Otherwise, infection is controlled by:
    (a) natural resistance and
    (b) good blood supply providing plenty of white cells and anti-bodies. This results in rapid repair.

16. The individual's resistance to disease

17. The tetanus organisms–they release toxins from the local site of injury which lead to muscular contractions of distant muscles e.g. of the masseter muscles

18. The smallest type of micro-organism–measured in millionths of a millimetre

19. They infect a body cell diverting its function to supporting the virus, thus enabling the latter to multiply and invade neighbouring cells

20. Hepatitis B; herpes ulcers, 'cold sores'; AIDS; herpetic whitlow

21. Passing of pathogenic micro-organisms from one person to another

22. (a) Those who have received large amounts of blood or blood products in the past six months
    (b) People who have suffered from jaundice in the last six months
    (c) Injecting drug addicts
    (d) Homosexuals
    (e) People from South-East Asia, sub-Saharan Africa, Eastern Mediterranean countries etc.

23. (a) *Streptococcus mutans*
    (b) Lactobacilli
    (c) Spirochaetes and anaerobes
    (d) A fungus–*Candida*

24. A thick creamy-yellow liquid resulting from localized inflammation. It contains white cells (dead and dying), organisms (dead and living), and necrotic (dead) tissue cells

25. An abscess

26. Serum hepatitis

27. What are the principles in the treatment of infection?
28. What are the possible outcomes of acute infection?
29. Why do plasma and white cells pass into tissues in acute inflammation?
30. What is a chronic inflammatory reaction?
31. Why might a patient produce a chronic inflammatory reaction rather than an acute inflammatory reaction?
32. What is a cyst?
33. What is meant by the term 'necrosis'?
34. What is a tumour?
35. Give the names of the two main types of tumour. Briefly state their main differences
36. What is meant by the following:
    (a) hypertrophy
    (b) hyperplasia
    (c) atrophy

27. (a) Remove the cause directly e.g. by extraction of a tooth, or indirectly e.g. by antibiotics
(b) Ensure good health

28. (a) Repair when the cause is removed or overcome
(b) Suppuration–formation of pus
(c) Extension into adjacent tissues, more rarely to a much wider area
(d) May become chronic

29. Plasma–to dilute the cause and to carry antibodies and antitoxins to the site.
White cells–to attack and try to destroy the cause

30. The reaction of the body to longstanding injury; often a 'walling off' type of tissue response

31. The patient's defence response may be high and/or the cause may be very mild

32. An abnormal cavity in the body. This cavity is lined and usually has semi-solid or fluid contents. Often develops from a chronic irritation

33. Cell death

34. An abnormal growth of tissue, serving no useful purpose, and which continues to grow at the expense of the surrounding tissues

35. Benign–slow growing, localized, harmless
Malignant–fast growing, initially localized, later having widespread metastases to other parts of the body, often fatal

36. (a) Increase in size of tissue due to enlargement of cells
(b) Increase in size of tissue due to the increased number of cells
(c) Reduction in size of tissue due to reduction in cell size or to a decreased number of cells

Sterilization

Questions

1. Define the following words:
   (a) sterilization
   (b) disinfection
   (c) antisepsis
   (d) commensal
2. What should an DA do with used dental instruments when the patient leaves the surgery?
3. What duties should the DA carry out to prepare the surgery for the next patient?
4. What are the risks associated with the cleaning of instruments?
5. How can these risks be kept to a minimum?
6. Why should instruments be rendered physically clean before final sterilization?
7. Which sterilization methods can spoil the temper of metal instruments?
8. How does debris on instruments affect sterilization?
9. What is the minimum amount of blood necessary to pass infection?
10. Which medical conditions are regarded as 'inoculation-risk' conditions?

Answers

1. (a) Killing of all micro-organisms including spores–there are no degrees of sterilisation
    (b) Destruction of pathogenic organisms but spores may remain
    (c) Disinfection which does not harm living tissues
    (d) A micro-organism normally present in the body which only causes disease if the balance between virulence and resistance is altered

2. Clean off all debris then sterilize

3. (a) All debris from the previous patient should be removed
    (b) Any equipment or surfaces which might have become contaminated with blood or saliva should be wiped down with an appropriate antiseptic
    (c) Hands must be washed and then the appropriate sterile instruments etc. are laid out

4. Spread of infection by:
    (a) contamination of or injury to DA
    (b) contamination of cleaning area and tools e.g. brush

5. (a) The DA should wear undamaged household gloves which must be washed with antiseptic after each use
    (b) Reduce splatter by use of soft cleaner e.g. paper and keep instruments well down in the sink
    (c) Dispose of soft cleaner immediately
    (d) If a brush needs to be used then at the least it should be disinfected after use
    (e) With a high-risk case 'sterilize' instruments to reduce the risk before any cleaning, then resterilize

6. (a) Contaminants may prevent true sterilization
    (b) Contaminants may be more difficult to remove after sterilization

7. (a) Direct heat
    (b) Dry heat at too high a temperature

8. (a) It can insulate the micro-organisms so that a lethal temperature is not reached
    (b) Protein matter can inactivate chemicals

9. One lymphocyte

10. Hepatitis B, AIDS, AIDS related syndrome. People with antibodies to human immuno-deficiency virus (HIV) are also considered in this category since they may eventually develop AIDS

11. What is the special risk when caring for these patients?
12. What are the disadvantages of chemical solutions for sterilizing?
13. How do strong chemical solutions affect micro-organisms?
14. Which groups of chemicals can kill viruses?
15. Name two commercial methods of sterilizing disposable items
16. Why is flaming not a suitable method for sterilizing metal instruments?
17. Why should the door of an autoclave not be opened during sterilization?
18. After sterilization, instruments removed from the sterilizer can easily become unsterile. How can this be prevented?
19. How would you dispose of the following:
    (a) scalpel blade?
    (b) highly infected waste?
    (c) used swabs?
    (d) waste amalgam?
20. How should a spillage of blood be dealt with?
21. After evacuating pus from an abscess how would you clean and prepare the suction apparatus ready for the next patient?
22. Why is it inadvisable to dispose of sharps in the general waste?

11. The conditions are transmitted via blood

12. (a) Many are not fully effective
    (b) To be effective they are highly poisonous
    (c) The length of time required to achieve sterilization
    (d) Damage to equipment and metal instruments from chemical corrosion

13. Mainly by damaging the cell wall

14. Aldehydes and hypochlorites freshly made and in adequate strength

15. (a) Gamma radiation
    (b) Ethylene oxide

16. They may become brittle

17. (a) Steam at high pressure is dangerous
    (b) The cycle will have to start again to be completed

18. (a) Leaving in sterilization bags or boxes
    (b) Immediate sterile transfer to sterile storage containers

19. (a) In a 'sharps' box or similar safe disposal container
    (b) Taking care not to spread infection; by placing in yellow plastic bag to warn everyone of dangerous contents, then sending for incineration
    (c) They are likely to be infected so care needs to be taken but ordinary disposal into waste bin should be adequate
    (d) Under water or potassium permanganate solution in container with well-fitting lid

20. All blood should be regarded as infected
    (a) Confine–cover by dropping paper towels on to spillage
    (b) Put on gloves, carefully transfer paper to plastic waste bag
    (c) Either soak the affected area with hypochlorite or aldehyde solution for at least 10 minutes or an alternative is to sprinkle area with hypochlorite-releasing granules e.g. Presept which react with the blood and can be wiped up after 10 minutes.If surface would be damaged by hypochlorite, cover with paper towels soaked in 2% aldehyde solution.
    (d) Wash and dry surface thoroughly

21. (a) Infected suction tip–careful disposal, or if non-disposable wash through with disinfectant then autoclave or dry-heat sterilize
    (b) Suction tube–suck through non-foaming disinfectant
    (c) Bottle–now containing disinfectant, empty down toilet then rinse with more antiseptic, finally a water rinse

22. There is a risk that refuse collectors may injure themselves or that scavengers on waste tips may sustain injury

23. How would you sterilize the following:
   (a) stock metal impression tray?
   (b) local anaesthetic needle?
   (c) general anaesthetic mask?
   (d) paper points?

24. Why should oral surgery burs be sterilized before use?

23. (a) Any standard sterilization method
  (b) Re-use not advised therefore do not sterilize
  (c) Not possible without special equipment so rely on disinfection e.g. soak in 2% aldehyde solution for 30 minutes then rinse thoroughly
  (d) Unused points in an autoclave with a drying cycle or in a dry heat sterilizer preferably on a lower temperature cycle

24. (a) They will be used in an open wound
  (b) If used to remove bone they could introduce infection into bone which can be difficult to overcome and is a very painful condition for the patient

Health and safety

Questions

1. Who is responsible for health and safety at work?
2. In relation to the Health and Safety at Work Act, what should you do if an accident at work occurs?
3. List the main groups of potential hazards to the DA in the surgery
4. List the types of potential non-dental hazards to patients and staff in a dental practice and give some examples
5. How can DAs protect themselves from chemical injury?
6. What action should be taken in the event of a chemical injury?
7. Give two ways in which mercury can be a danger to the dental team
8. What are the symptoms of mercury poisoning?
9. Indicate the area of skin most likely to absorb mercury
10. List the major potential sources of mercury vapour

Answers

1. Everyone–employer, staff, also manufacturers and suppliers

2. (a) Render first aid
   (b) Take action to prevent an immediate recurrence
   (c) Report the accident to your employer and make a note in the accident book. Report even if no injury or damage so that safety procedures are reviewed.

3. (a) Infection–general–e.g. common cold, tuberculosis etc
      oral–cross-infection from instruments etc
      infected fragments of tooth, calculus, etc.
      dental aerosol being inhaled or drifting into eyes
   (b) Physical injury from sharp instruments, flying debris
   (c) Chemical injury e.g. hypochlorite and glutaraldehyde solutions
   (d) Noxious vapours e.g. acrylic monomer fumes
   (e) Mercury
   (f) X-radiation
   (g) Anaesthetic gases
   (h) Fire e.g. from gas burner

4. (a) General mechanical and physical e.g. state of the entrance, floors, stairs etc, obstructions, poor lighting.
   (b) Equipment–insecure, unstable etc
   (c) Electrical e.g. faulty plugs, insulation or trailing cables
   (d) Fire–naked flames, cigarettes, inflammable liquids

5. (a) Put on sound household gloves and protective apron before handling strong chemicals
   (b) Eye protection should be worn
   (c) Follow manufacturers' instructions

6. (a) First aid–copious washing with water and apply antidote
   (b) Prevention–warn to stop other people being injured
   (c) Report the accident

7. (a) Contact through skin
   (b) Inhalation of vapour

8. Irritability, metallic taste, increased salivation, kidney disorders, neurological changes

9. The hands, especially stagnant areas such as under nails

10. (a) Spillage–especially if it is incompletely cleared up
    (b) Waste amalgam
    (c) Around an amalgamator
    (d) From faulty seals of amalgam capsules–mainly if re-used

11. How can mercury hazard in the surgery be reduced?

12. How can a surgery be checked for mercury contamination?

13. How may nitrous oxide and halothane be a danger to surgery and theatre staff?

14. List the main potential sources of anaesthetic gas pollution

15. How might hepatitis B virus be transmitted in the surgery?

16. Briefly, what is the role of the DA in helping to prevent transmission of hepatitis B from known-risk patients?

17. What is the hazard of X-radiation?

18. What is the simplest way to reduce X-radiation hazard in the surgery?

19. What signs could indicate that an X-ray machine was not safe?

11. (a) By avoiding spillage e.g. place amalgamator on a plastic or foil tray before filling mercury reservoir
    (b) Keep mercury and waste amalgam under water in sealed container
    (c) Well-ventilated room
    (d) Do not handle, wear gloves if risk of contact. No open-toed shoes

12. (a) Visually for tiny droplets in crevices etc.
    (b) Commercially available powders and discs to indicate the presence of mercury vapour
    (c) Electronic 'sniffers' are available through Health Authorities

13. (a) Toxic–liver damage, spontaneous abortion
    (b) Soporific–staff become drowsy if inadequate ventilation or scavenging

14. (a) Leaks from the anaesthetic machine
    (b) Escape from an ill-fitting mask
    (c) Exhaled by the patient

15. Blood contamination is the most likely method, although saliva can carry the virus
    (a) Directly–patient's blood to staff wound e.g. 'needlestick' injuries
    (b) Indirectly via contaminated instruments breaking the skin of a member of staff
    (c) Incompletely sterilized instrument damaging staff or another patient.
    Up to 4% of UK population have had hepatitis B. There are an estimated 600,000 carriers, many unaware that they are carriers.

16. (a) When making appointments make sure that infection-risk patients are booked in at a suitable time and that the special nature of the appointment is clearly marked in the book
    (b) Proper preparation of the surgery
    (c) Full personal precautions
    (d) Care when assisting not to spread contamination around the surgery
    (e) To follow sterilization and clean-up procedures
    (f) Any items being taken from the surgery e.g. impressions and waste must be properly cared for and labelled 'danger of infection' for the protection of other persons

17. It can cause cell damage and even death of cells

18. Keep the machine switched off except when in use

19. (a) Warm X-ray head
    (b) Oil leaks from X-ray head–these should be reported immediately.

20. Why are the dental team particularly at risk from X-radiation?
21. How can the radiation risk to the DA be kept to a minimum?
22. List the main causes of eye damage likely to be suffered by the dental team.
23. How can eye injuries be prevented?
24. What are the signs and symptoms of eye damage?
25. What is the treatment for eye damage?
26. Why should care be taken in the use of restorative curing lights?
27. Give the reasons for maintaining a well-ventilated surgery.
28. What is a 'dental aerosol' and what is it likely to contain?
29. How can possible problems arising from dental aerosol be reduced?

20. Because of the number of films which are taken. If the correct procedures are followed the risk should not be increased

21. If the DA needs to be present when films are being taken then:
   (a) Do not stand in path of the main beam, preferably to one side
   (b) Stand at least 2 metres from the tube, which must not be held
   (c) Stand behind a protective wall or screen or wear a lead apron
   (d) Use film holders if possible but if not, then patient (or parent wearing another lead apron) should hold the film
   (e) Switch off the machine after use
   (f) Use a radiation monitoring system

22. Penetrating, infective or allergic
   (a) Injury e.g. from flying debris
   (b) Chemicals mainly from contact with hand contamination
   (c) Cross-infection either bacterial or viral

23. (a) Goggles or glasses should be worn when there is a possible risk
   (b) Posture–leaning close to the patient increases the hazard
   (c) Suction–efficient use of high-volume suction reduces the spread of oral debris

24. Those of acute inflammation, especially loss of function

25. (a) Irrigation–immediate and copious washing with water
   (b) Medical attention for all blunt injuries and for infection which does not clear within 24 hours

26. These lights have been associated with eye problems and so care in their use is advisable. Do not look directly at the light tip. Wear protective glasses, not sunglasses. If a light shield is available make sure it is fitted ready for use

27. Reduction of pollution including:
   (a) Microbial–general and oral
   (b) Vapours and fumes–mercury, acrylic monomer, anaesthetic gases

28. (a) A mist spray arising from the use of certain dental equipment e.g. air turbine, triple syringe, ultrasonic scaler
   (b) (i) water and saliva; (ii) bacteria and viruses; (iii) food debris, plaque and calculus; (iv) tooth and filling material particles

29. (a) Prevention–air conditioning with a fresh air intake
      –efficient high-volume suction exhausting to the exterior
   (b) Surgery cleaning–thorough and regular cleaning including damp dusting
   (c) Personal protection–separate surgery clothes, laundered daily
      –cleansing of exposed skin and hair
   (d) Special protection–protective glasses, face mask changed regularly

Radiography

Questions

1. What is X-radiation?
2. What are the genetic effects of radiation on the body?
3. Which types of cells are more sensitive to the harmful effects of radiation?
4. Give examples of the damage which may occur
5. What are the two main uses of X-radiation in medicine?
6. Why should the X-ray machine be switched off when not in use?
7. How can DAs check whether they are receiving dangerous radiation?
8. Where are the safe places for a DA during the taking of an X-ray film?
9. Where should a film monitor badge be worn and why in that position?
10. Why is it preferable not to take X-ray films during pregnancy?
11. What precautions can be taken to protect patients during radiography?
12. Name three types of intra-oral film
13. What is a radiograph?
14. How should dental X-ray films be stored?
15. Why is lead foil included in the dental film packet?
16. What is the main use of a dental periapical film?
17. What special care should be taken when loading extra-oral film cassettes?
18. Name the standard lateral skull radiograph taken for orthodontic assessment
19. What is the effect of X-rays on an X-ray film?

Answers

1. It is part of the electromagnetic spectrum possessing short penetrating rays–shorter than ultraviolet light

2. Affect chromosomes leading to mutations and abnormalities e.g. handicapping conditions

3. Reproductive tissue, embryos, blood cells, epithelium

4. Sterility, premature death, leukaemia, dermatitis ranging from redness through to ulceration

5. (a) Diagnostic
   (b) Therapeutic–treatment by the controlled killing of cells e.g. cancer. This is called radiotherapy

6. In case a fault does develop, radiation will be kept to a minimum

7. By wearing a film monitor which is processed at regular intervals

8. (a) To the side or behind the path of the main beam and at least 2 metres away
   (b) Better still is to stand behind a protective screen, if there is one

9. At or below waist level. Monitoring radiation received at gonad level

10. The risk is of radiation damage to the developing embryo

11. (a) Use of a lead apron placed over the patient's trunk
    (b) Use of fast film and therefore short exposure time
    (c) Use the minimum number of films
    (d) Avoidance of retakes

12. Periapical, bite-wing, occlusal

13. A fully processed X-ray film

14. In a dry cool dark place away from radiation and fumes. Oldest films available for first use

15. (a) To absorb radiation which has passed through teeth and bone
    (b) To protect the film from back-scatter radiation

16. To produce a picture of a tooth plus the surrounding tissues

17. (a) Load only in the dark or under a correctly filtered light
    (b) Hands and all surfaces must be dry
    (c) Check previous film removed from cassette
    (d) Touch film edges or corners only
    (e) Avoid contamination or damage to intensifying screens

18. Lateral cephalograph

19. Silver salts in the emulsion of the film undergo change when exposed to X-radiation. The lighter parts of the radiograph have received less radiation

20. List four factors which affect the exposure time of intra-oral films
21. What is used to keep the exposure time of extra-oral films to a minimum?
22. Why do metal fillings appear white on radiographs?
23. What can a dental surgeon learn from a bite-wing radiograph?
24. Which teeth are usually visible on an oblique lateral radiograph?
25. What hard structures are shown on a dental panoramic radiograph?

Processing

26. How can the DA reduce the amount of radiation received by a patient?
27. Why can X-ray films be opened 'safely' under a safelight?
28. What is on the surface of a dental X-ray film?
29. Before starting the developing process for a batch of films in the darkroom,what procedures must the DA observe?
30. With an automatic film processor what are the duties of the DA?
31. Why should films be agitated in the developer?

20. (a) Density of tissue
    (b) Thickness of overlying tissue
    (c) X-ray tube to film distance
    (d) Speed of the film

21. Intensifying screens which enhance the radiation and reduce exposure time

22. The metal absorbs X-rays, preventing them from reaching the film. As a result no changes take place in the silver salts on the film in that area. Radiation is absorbed less by enamel and dentine which show as shades of grey on the radiograph.

23. (a) Presence and extent of interproximal and occlusal caries
    (b) Some information about existing restorations e.g. leakage at the gingival margins
    (c) Presence of interdental calculus
    (d) The state of the crests of bone between the teeth

24. The cheek teeth, that is the premolars and molars

25. Maxilla, mandible, the teeth

Processing

26. Avoidance of retakes by:
    (a) Correct processing of films
    (b) Correct identification of radiographs
    (c) Careful filing and storage of radiographs

27. The special glass filter permits the passage of light at a wavelength which does not affect films during the short time they are open in the dark room

28. Silver halide salts in emulsion

29. Check the following:
    (a) correct volume and temperature of developing and fixing solutions
    (b) timer is available
    (c) safelight is working
    (d) availability of film hangers
    (e) name recording system available
    (f) film names transferred to recording system
    (g) dark room is light-proof

30. Daily—on arrival check fluid levels, if satisfactory then switch on. At regular intervals—replace solutions, clean interior etc. as advised by the manufacturer

31. (a) To dislodge any surface air bubbles
    (b) To make sure films do not stick together

32. Why should spots of developer or fixer be washed off skin or clothes immediately?

33. Give five most important aspects of dark room processing

34. Why is it necessary for films to stay in the developer for an accurately measured length of time?

35. Why are films washed in water following their removal from the developer?

36. Give four reasons why films are placed in the fixing solution

37. What may be the processing reasons for these faulty radiographs?
(a) only part of the film processed?
(b) dark image?
(c) spots on radiograph?
(d) no image?
(e) emulsion stripping?

38. Give at least five reasons why a radiograph may be fogged

39. Why should radiographs be dried before filing away?

40. Why should radiographs be stored?

41. What is the legal time to retain radiographs?

32. To reduce the chance of dermatitis or staining of the clothes

33. (a) No unwanted light
(b) Correct identification of films at all stages
(c) Use of solutions in the correct order
(d) Correct timing
(e) Proper washing and drying

34. To allow for the complete chemical changes of the crystals in the film emulsion which will produce the best possible picture.

35. To remove developer agents and so prevent contamination of the fixing solution. This will also prevent 'fogging'.

36. (a) To dissolve out crystals in the emulsion which have not undergone change due to radiation. Leaving them would lead to discoloration
(b) To neutralize the chemical reaction on the film
(c) To produce a visible image
(d) To harden the emulsion

37. (a) Film not covered by solutions, films in contact during developing
(b) Over developed–temperature too high, time too long, solution too strong
(c) Chemical splashes, moisture penetration
(d) Fixer first
(e) Hot water used for washing

38. (a) Adverse storage conditions
(b) Exposure to extraneous radiation
(c) Old films
(d) Exposure to white light
(e) Faulty safelight
(f) Wrong safelight filter
(g) Excessively long development
(h) Development at very high temperatures
(i) Exhausted developer
(j) Inadequate washing before placing in fixer

39. If filed damp, the surface may be damaged and useful information be lost

40. (a) For reference
   (i) when treating the patient during the current course of treatment
   (ii) at subsequent courses of treatment to review the earlier state of the hard tissues of the mouth
(b) As a legal requirement

41. Six years

Prevention of dental disease

Questions

1. What is the meaning of
   (a) primary prevention
   (b) secondary prevention?
2. What five local factors can lead to gingival inflammation?
3. Give the main factors associated with the development of dental caries?
4. How are teeth cleaned naturally?
5. What is the name given to the surface film which adheres to hard tissues in the mouth?
6. What is the importance of pellicle?
7. Define dental plaque.
8. List the constituents of plaque.
9. What harmful substances are formed by plaque?
10. How can patients clearly demonstrate their plaque?
11. Give some other methods used in the surgery to demonstate plaque to patients
12. What is the effect of retained plaque on the gingiva?
13. What is meant by a 'plaque index'?
14. What is a plaque index used for?
15. How long does it take for substantial amounts of plaque to collect?
16. Briefly state how plaque forms
17. Why are the acids of plaque considered to be harmful?
18. Why are the toxins of plaque considered to be harmful?

Answers

1. (a) Preventing disease before it starts
   (b) Detection and treatment of disease and prevention of recurrence

2. (a) Plaque
   (b) Calculus
   (c) Poorly aligned teeth
   (d) Poorly finished restorations
   (e) Ill-fitting dentures or orthodontic appliances

3. (a) Diet–high in carbohydrate and sucrose
           –high intake of acidic items e.g. citrus fruit, fizzy drinks
   (b) Frequent between-meals snacks
   (c) Plaque retention
   (d) Poor tooth shape and structure

4. By the action of the tongue, lips and cheeks, and saliva

5. Pellicle. It forms less easily on highly polished surfaces such as porcelain crowns

6. Dental plaque develops on the pellicle

7. A complex film of oral material which adheres to the teeth

8. Water, bacteria, carbohydrate, bacterial waste products, mucin

9. (a) Acids
   (b) Toxins

10. By use of disclosing agents

11. By polishing some of the teeth and comparing with the dull surface of adjacent plaque-covered teeth. Use of fluorescent dye and a Plaklight

12. It causes inflammation.

13. A system of assessing the amount of plaque present on teeth

14. To show change in plaque control and so indicate to the patient improvement or otherwise

15. Less than 48 hours

16. Pellicle re-forms soon after cleaning, oral bacteria become attached (with the aid of mucin) to the pellicle and multiply

17. If left in contact with the enamel they cause decalcification

18. Left in contact with the periodontal tissues they are irritants and cause inflammation

19. How can dietary control assist in the prevention of dental disease?
20. What is meant by hidden sugars?
21. What is the effect of frequent citrus fruit or juice intake?
22. Why is it important for the expectant mother to have adequate calcium and vitamins in her diet?
23. How can a patient's food intake be assessed for quality?
24. What can we expect to learn from the information provided?
25. How does fluoride toothpaste help to prevent caries?
26. How may fluoride be taken by a child to be incorporated into the forming teeth?
27. What is the effect on the teeth of taking too many fluoride tablets for a prolonged period of time?
28. Despite using fluoride toothpaste some people still develop new carious cavities–give some reasons for this
29. What factors assist normal formation of bones and teeth?
30. What are the benefits of mouth brushing?
31. What are the important factors in selecting a new toothbrush?

19. (a) Type of food–control intake of carbohydrates–organisms in plaque convert refined carbohydrates to acid
    (b) Frequency–avoid snacks–since the acidity of plaque rises within five minutes of eating carbohydrate and declines over the next hour or so, frequent intake of snacks raises the acidity
    (c) Consistency–choose food carefully–sticky foods adhere to teeth longer and are more difficult to remove

20. Many foods and prepared meals, including savoury items, contain sucrose. Food labels should be checked.

21. This is very acid and erodes the enamel making it more susceptible to attack by caries

22. To assist the normal formatiom of bones and teeth of the foetus

23. By asking the patient to keep a diet sheet for 3 or 4 days.

24. (a) Frequency of eating and drinking
    (b) Intake of carbohydates as well as other types of food
    (c) Additional sugars e.g. amount added to drinks during each day
    (d) Hidden sugars
    (e) General balance or otherwise of the diet

25. (a) Some of the fluoride is absorbed into the outer enamel surface which makes it more resistant to acid attack
    (b) Bacteria appear to produce less acid in the presence of fluoride

26. (a) In the water supply
    (b) Fluoride tablets or drops
    (c) In milk
    (d) In salt (Switzerland)

27. The developing teeth could show white or brown markings called mottling

28. (a) A false sense of security develops and less emphasis is given to other preventive measures e.g. effective brushing, diet control
    (b) Fluoride in toothpastes can only affect the dentine by entry through the carious cavity and so has a limited effect

29. Adequate calcium and vitamins A and D in the diet and adequate fluoride taken during the formation of teeth

30. (a) Removal of plaque
    (b) Gum stimulation

31. (a) Size–a short head is preferable
    (b) Texture–medium or soft nylon multi-tufted, unless advised otherwise by the dental surgeon or hygienist
    (c) Shape–straight handle with flat brushing surface except for special situations

32. What are the disadvantages of large toothbrushes?

33. How may patients clean their teeth apart from the use of a toothbrush?

34. Toothpastes contain certain amounts of detergent and abrasive material and are alkaline. What is the purpose of each constituent?

35. Why is it important to clean the teeth properly after the last food and drink at night?

36. How can the patient be shown areas of the mouth which are not being cleaned properly?

37. When should dentures and orthodontic appliances be cleaned?

38. Why should dentures and appliances be cleaned regularly?

39. How does saliva help to reduce dental disease?

40. What tooth brushing advice is usually given by the dental surgeon to patients whose gums bleed?

41. In what three ways can the dental surgeon reduce the incidence of fissure caries?

32. (a) General difficulty in manipulation
    (b) Difficult to clean individual teeth
    (c) Do not get into spaces where teeth are missing
    (d) Special difficulty in cleaning buccal to upper wisdom teeth
    (e) Possibly damage the sulci and tissue at the end of each quadrant

33. (a) Eating fibrous foods
    (b) Vigorous mouth rinsing or use of irrigation machine e.g. Water-Pik
    (c) Use of tongue
    (d) Use of dental floss
    (e) Use of wood points
    (f) Use of chemical agents e.g. sodium bicarbonate

34. (a) Detergent, for removal of animal and vegetable fats and oils
    (b) Abrasives, to remove stains
    (c) Alkaline, to help neutralize plaque acids

35. So that a minimal amount of plaque remains on the teeth overnight. During sleep:
    (a) salivary flow is reduced so that oral acids are less diluted
    (b) plaque remains undisturbed, by tongue and food, thus there can be prolonged attack on the dental tissues

36. Using a disclosing solution or tablet, residual plaque is stained red or blue. Using a large mirror the patient can then be shown the stained areas and the significance explained.

37. After each meal–rinsing if brushing is not possible
    Last thing at night–it is preferable to leave dentures out overnight

38. (a) Food debris and plaque collect around clasps and wires which if left cause disease in adjacent tissues
    (b) Debris and plaque also collects on the mucosal surface of the acrylic which if left can lead to inflammation and fungal infection

39. (a) It helps to wash away debris
    (b) It is slightly alkaline and helps to neutralize acids
    (c) It contains antibacterial substances

40. After checking for possible hormonal or medical causes; to continue to brush, but carefully and thoroughly, and using the correct textured toothbrush and correct method. Most gingivitis is due to plaque

41. (a) Fissure sealants
    (b) Prophylactic occlusal fissure amalgams
    (c) Application of topical fluoride

Periodontology

Questions

1. What is periodontology?
2. What is the most common disease of periodontal tissues?
3. In Britain, how often is this condition likely to affect:
   (a) 15–19-year-olds
   (b) 30–40-year-old persons?
4. Among which groups of people is it more likely to be found?
5. Which tissues make up the periodontal tissues?
6. How deep is a normal gingival sulcus?
7. What is gingivitis?
8. What are the symptoms of chronic gingivitis?
9. What are the signs of chronic gingivitis?
10. What is meant by false pocketing?
11. Why are the gingiva in gingivitis redder than usual?
12. Define 'periodontitis'
13. Where does periodontal disease usually start?
14. What are the signs and symptoms of chronic periodontal disease?
15. What is a periodontal pocket?
16. How is the depth of a pocket assessed?
17. How is the mobility of teeth assessed?
18. What types of radiograph are taken as part of the assessment of patients with periodontal disease?
19. For what reasons are these radiographs taken?
20. Give the main causative factor in periodontal disease
21. What other main factors help to cause periodontal disease?

Answers

1. The study of the prevention and treatment of diseases of the periodontal tissues

2. Chronic periodontal disease

3. (a) 50%
   (b) 95%

4. (a) Males
   (b) Lower socio-economic groups
   More than anything this reflects lack of motivation towards oral hygiene.

5. Gingiva, cementum, periodontal ligament and supporting bone

6. 1–2 mm

7. Inflammation of the gingiva

8. Mainly bleeding on brushing but halitosis and pain can occur

9. Rounded swollen shiny appearance with a zone of redness at the margin

10. Inflammed gingiva are swollen; this creates a deeper gingival crevice above the amelo-cemental junction than usual and is called a false pocket

11. Due to the inflammatory process there is an increased blood supply

12. Inflammation of the periodontal tissues, especially the ligament

13. At the gingival margin as gingivitis

14. Those of gingivitis plus detachment of the interdental papillae, pocketing, gingival recession, loss of alveolar supporting bone, tooth mobility, tilting or drifting of teeth, possibly pain

15. Where the gingival attachment to the tooth has moved apically from the amelo-cemental junction

16. With a pocket measuring probe

17. The movement of the crown in a bucco-lingual direction measured in millimetres. Class 1 is less than 1 mm, class 2 is 1–2 mm etc

18. Periapicals give most detail, a panoramic radiograph gives an overall view

19. To determine the state of the teeth and the supporting tissues

20. Bacterial plaque

21. Anything which inhibits plaque removal e.g. poor contour of the teeth or of the dental arch, calculus, ledges on restorations, partial dentures

22. List the factors necessary for oral bacteria to flourish.

23. Which factor determines the severity of periodontal disease?

24. Give three consequences of having an unopposed tooth.

25. What can be the consequences on the surrounding teeth of loss of one tooth?

26. Give examples of how patients can inflict injuries to their gingiva.

27. When does breathing affect the gums harmfully?

28. How may orthodontic treatment lead to gingival disease?

29. Give examples of drugs and chemicals which have harmful effects on the gingiva.

30. What is pregnancy gingivitis?

31. How may gingivitis encourage further gingival disease?

32. How does calculus lead to further periodontal disease?

33. What is a periodontal abscess?

34. How does a periodontal abscess develop?

35. Acute ulcerative gingivitis leads to damage of which particular area of gingival tissue?

22. Nutrients, mineral salts, optimum oxygen concentration and an energy source such as glucose

23. The amount of plaque, that is the degree of cleaning

24. (a) Increased plaque and calculus
    (b) Greater chance of periodontal disease
    (c) Over-eruption of the tooth

25. (a) Drifting of teeth on either side. This leads to loss of contact points and to pocketing
    (b) Over-eruption of the opposing tooth. This can lead to pocketing around that tooth
    (c) Increased usage of other teeth e.g. using other side of the mouth

26. (a) Vigorous tooth brushing
    (b) A hard brush and a horizontal brushing technique
    (c) Using finger nails, pins etc

27. People who mouth breathe often have reduced lubrication of the gingiva which increases the effect of plaque as its products are not diluted

28. (a) Removable appliances not regularly removed for cleaning
    (b) Interdental spacing not cleaned
    (c) Inadequate cleaning around fixed appliances

29. Epanutin prescribed for epileptics. Drugs which reduce salivation e.g. some antidepressants

30. Because of hormonal changes the gingival reaction to plaque is exaggerated. Careful but thorough hygiene usually controls the condition which normally resolves itself after the birth

31. (a) Bleeding and pain discourage the patient from cleaning
    (b) Swelling of the gingiva leads to pockets which are difficult to clean

32. Plaque forms on the subgingival surface of the calculus–toxins released by the bacteria irritate the pocket walls leading to increased inflammation

33. Localized acute inflammation of the periodontal tissues resulting in pus formation. A periapical abscess is usually of pulpal origin

34. Infection in the pocket may become more severe or the normal pocket drainage be interrupted leading to a build-up of pus

35. The interdental papillae. They become ulcerated and appear saucer-shaped

36. Give at least four important features of acute ulcerative gingivitis

37. What three measures may the patient be asked to carry out in the treatment of acute ulcerative gingivitis?

38. Define the word 'prognosis'

39. Give the objective of the primary phase of periodontal treatment

40. How can this objective be achieved?

41. What are the main problems for patients in achieving optimum plaque control?

42. What methods can patients use to reduce plaque in their mouths?

43. Which tooth surfaces are most difficult to clean?

44. What equipment for interdental cleaning is available to patients?

45. Why is careful instruction in their use most important?

46. One method of brushing is to 'brush the way the tooth grows'–what are the advantages of this method?

47. What are the advantages of the 'miniscrub' method?

48. Faulty tooth brushing can damage which three tissues?

49. How can the DA help patients to improve their plaque control?

50. Give the role of antiseptic mouthwashes in maintaining oral hygiene

36. (a) Swollen gums
   (b) Gums bleed easily
   (c) Pain
   (d) Foul smell
   (e) Grey dead tissue on the gum surface
   (f) Ulcerated interdental papillae
   (g) Enlarged lymphatic nodes
   (h) Temperature sometimes raised

37. (a) Take metronidazole tablets or antibiotics
   (b) Frequent oxygen-releasing mouthwashes. The causative organisms are anaerobes
   (c) Very gentle but thorough tooth and gum cleaning

38. The expected course of a disease and a prediction of the outcome with treatment

39. To resolve reversible disease

40. By removal of causative factors especially plaque

41. Time, dexterity, tooth anatomy

42. Thorough cleaning of all surfaces of tooth crowns using suitable aids

43. Interdental, mesial and distal

44. (a) Dental floss or tape
   (b) Interdental wood points
   (c) Interdental brushes such as interproximal or bottle types

45. (a) The interdental tissues can be damaged
   (b) To try to ensure that they are used effectively

46. (a) Helps to remove debris from the interdental space
   (b) Reduces cervical tooth and gingival abrasion

47. (a) Patient is encouraged to brush a small number of teeth at a time
   (b) The gingival crevices are cleaned

48. Gingivae, cementum, dentine

49. Following instruction from the dental surgeon
   (a) Teach the patient how to disclose
   (b) Help the patient to understand oral hygiene instructions
   (c) Observe cleaning technique to highlight strong and weak points

50. (a) They help to remove gross debris
   (b) Some bacteria are killed
   (c) After surgery when brushing may not be advisable

51. How does diet help to maintain healthy gums?

52. How can recurrence of periodontal disease be prevented?

53. In what ways can patients help to reduce the severity of periodontal disease?

54. What is the main reason for carrying out periodontal surgery?

55. List the most commonly performed periodontal surgical procedures

51. (a) Eating a balanced healthy diet helps to maintain good general health
    (b) Friction of food can help but is not an alternative to proper oral hygiene procedures

52. Removal of causative factors particularly plaque. The patient is mainly responsible for prevention once the dental surgeon has attended to the other causes

53. (a) Maintain a high standard of oral hygiene
    (b) Regular dental checks

54. To help the patient to carry out good plaque control by improving tissue contour and by removing unhealthy tissue

55. (a) Simple pocketing–subgingival curettage, gingivectomy
    (b) Deeper pocketing–flap operations

Calculus

Questions

1. Define dental calculus
2. How can calculus be detected?
3. What covers the outer surface of calculus?
4. Name the two types of calculus
5. What is the importance of saliva in the formation of calculus?
6. Why is calculus in a periodontal pocket dark in colour?
7. In which particular areas is supragingival calculus found?
8. Why is it found there?
9. Why does subgingival calculus collect progressively in an apical direction?
10. Why does calculus form mainly behind the lower incisor teeth?
11. Briefly state what happens to the periodontal tissues as subgingival calculus continues to accumulate

Answers

1. Mineralized plaque–mainly calcium and magnesium salts
2. Visually, by probing or from radiographs
3. Plaque
4. Supragingival and subgingival
5. The mineral salts come from the saliva
6. Gingival bleeding leads to blood breakdown products which are incorporated into the forming calculus
7. Lingual to lower incisors and buccal to upper first permanent molars
8. Saliva ducts are adjacent to these areas
9. Plaque on the gingival surface is in a stagnation area and cannot be removed with a toothbrush; it becomes calcified increasing apically.
10. (a) 70% of saliva comes from the submandibular gland
    (b) It is not an easy place for patients to clean properly
    (c) As a result mineralization of plaque easily occurs
11. (a) Gingival inflammation continues with swelling and bleeding
    (b) Stagnation occurs with further plaque retention
    (c) All the periodontal tissues become inflammed and fibres are destroyed
    (d) The inflammatory process spreads to involve the supporting bone and leads to bone loss. Initially the interdental bone crest is damaged, but later the socket wall becomes involved, leading to tooth mobility.

Scaling

Questions

1. What are the objectives of scaling teeth?
2. List the methods used to remove calculus
3. Give the types of instruments available to remove calculus
4. Why are teeth polished after scaling?
5. What are the risks to patients during polishing?
6. What instruments are used to polish teeth?
7. Why might local anaesthesia be required for scaling?
8. Which types of patients need special precautions to be taken before deep scaling is carried out?
9. What is meant by 'root planning'?
10. Why is root planning carried out?
11. What are the potential hazards to the DA when assisting with scaling or when handling scaling instruments?

Answers

1. To remove all calculus and plaque in order to produce a smooth surface for better plaque control

2. Hand, ultrasonic or sonic scaling

3. (a) Hand–sickle, curette and hoes of various designs
   (b) Ultrasonic–inserts similar in design to scalers
   (c) Sonic–special types of bur

4. To produce a smooth surface and remove staining

5. (a) Polishing paste getting into their eyes
   (b) Inhalation or ingestion of polishing cup or brush if not properly locked into the handpiece or a mandrel

6. Small brushes or rubber cups in a slow-running handpiece; polishing strips

7. Scaling in deep pockets can cause pain to teeth or soft tissues

8. (a) Medical risk patients in particular those with rheumatic heart disease, heart valve problems, bleeding disorders, organ transplants, etc
   (b) Infection risk patients

9. The deep scaling of the roots of the teeth

10. (a) To remove calculus and plaque from the root surface
    (b) To remove bacterial toxins from cementum to encourage re-attachment of the periodontal ligament
    (c) Some cleaning of the soft tissue walls of the pocket also occurs

11. (a) Flying debris such as calculus
    (b) Aerosol debris from use of 3-in-1 syringe or ultrasonic scaling apparatus
    (c) Puncture wounds during cleaning of instruments

Caries

Questions

1. What is dental caries?
2. What components are necessary for dental caries?
3. What is the main micro-organism associated with caries?
4. What is the main causative factor in caries?
5. How does the main causative factor lead to caries?
6. Where are the common sites for dental caries to occur in the mouth, and why does it favour these sites?
7. Give at least three ways in which the dental surgeon may detect caries
8. Why is plaque an important factor in the caries process?
9. Why is plaque less common on the palatal surfaces of teeth?
10. What is the effect of saliva on the occurrence of caries?
11. Why are enamel fissures more prone to caries?
12. Why is enamel specially at risk in the hour after sucrose has been taken?
13. Why do most new carious lesions occur within six years of eruption of permanent teeth?
14. How is the initial lesion in enamel caries of a smooth surface recognized?

Answers

1. The demineralization and disintegration of hard tooth substance by acids produced by bacteria

2. A tooth, bacterial plaque and food substrate

3. *Streptococcus mutans*

4. Refined sugar (sucrose)

5. Refined sugar is metabolized by bacteria, the end-product is acid which decalcifies enamel

6. (a) Pits and fissures
   (b) Interproximal surfaces
   (c) The gingival region of the crown
   (d) Edges of defective restorations
   These are stagnation areas where plaque collects

7. (a) Visually without aids, i.e. an actual hole, or a change in tooth colour
   (b) Using mirror and probe
   (c) Bite-wing radiographs
   (d) Transillumination

8. It contains the bacteria and carbohydrate which lead to acid formation.

9. Because of the cleansing action of the tongue

10. (a) It helps to reduce the incidence of caries by
    (i) washing away food debris
    (ii) reducing the number of bacteria present
    (iii) diluting sugars and acids
    (b) It is slightly alkaline and helps to neutralize acids in the mouth
    Patients with a dry mouth from disease or therapy are more prone to caries and need more preventive care

11. It is difficult to remove plaque from these narrow stagnation areas, which are narrower than one toothbrush bristle

12. The pH of plaque is lowered (it becomes more acid) for at least one hour

13. (a) With children there is less control of intake of sugar and drinks
    (b) More notice is taken of dietary advice after experience of caries
    (c) Surfaces are less resistant until dietary and toothpaste fluoride has had time to be absorbed
    (d) The obvious sites for caries have not been filled

14. By a white opaque area

15. How does the operator produce a similar effect during one form of dental treatment?

16. What factors can lead to arrest of an early carious lesion?

17. What is meant by remineralization of teeth?

18. What are topical fluorides and in what forms are they available?

19. What is a 'sticky fissure'?

20. How is the decay process aided by the early lesion?

21. Give the advantages of early detection of a carious lesion

22. Give the common causes for carious lesions which occur at the gingival margins of teeth

23. When a cavity just involves dentine, patients often complain of pain with hot drinks and hot food. Why is this?

24. Why does an apparently small cavity sometimes turn out to be so large?

25. What is meant by secondary enamel caries?

26. Give the sources of secondary enamel caries

27. What is the probable result of secondary enamel caries?

28. Why does carious dentine become cheese-like?

29. How can the tooth itself delay the caries process from reaching the pulp?

15. During the primary stage of the acid-etch techniques

16. (a) Improved plaque control
(b) Control of sugar intake
(c) Topical fluoride

17. At the earliest stage of decalcification of enamel it is possible for the process to be reversed and for mineral salts to re-enter the enamel matrix. Probing to detect an early carious lesion can damage this matrix and prevent remineralization.

18. (a) Fluoride salts applied to the surface of the enamel
(b) Available as solutions, gels, varnish and toothpaste

19. An enamel fissure into which the point of a probe just enters and sticks. This may mean that the fissure is naturally wide and non-carious or it can be a sign of early caries

20. The roughened surface allows plaque to collect more easily

21. (a) Prevention and remineralization may be possible
(b) If restoration is necessary then only a small filling is needed
(c) Small restorations do not weaken the remaining tooth structure

22. (a) Inadequate cleaning leading to retained plaque
(b) Over-enthusiastic cleaning leading to abrasion

23. The layer of sound dentine is getting thin, so that there is easy conduction of heat through the tooth

24. Dentine caries can progress rapidly within the enamel shell and without necessarily involving further enamel caries

25. Enamel caries at the amelo–dentinal junction caused by dentine caries; thus it is caries spreading from the inside of the tooth but following initial entry through the enamel

26. The caries may be in a new cavity, remain after cavity preparation or originate from marginal leakage of an existing restoration

27. Enamel is destroyed from the amelo–dentinal junction. This destruction plus the undermining of the enamel by dentine caries leads to weak unsupported enamel which fractures easily and a large cavity can suddenly appear. This often encourages the patient to attend, perhaps in the belief that a filling has fallen out

28. The dentine caries process involves demineralization of the inorganic content and destruction (proteolysis) of the organic content. When this has occurred the remaining tooth substance is firm but soft enough to be removed with hand instruments

29. By laying down secondary dentine in the pulp chamber

30. Why is root caries often a rapid process?

31. At the end of cavity preparation which type of dental material can be applied to dentine to help arrest any residual early caries?

32. Why does an inflamed pulp cause pain?

33. In general terms give two main causes of pulp death

34. What may happen to an untreated periapical abscess?

35. How can the DA assist in the detection of caries?

30. (a) There is no enamel to slow the process
   (b) There are fewer mineral salts in cementum and dentine
   (c) The interdental root areas are difficult to clean

31. Calcium hydroxide.This is alkaline as well as containing calcium salts

32. The inflamatory exudate increases the pressure in the pulp chamber which stimulates the pulp nerve endings

33. (a) Trauma
   (b) Chronic irritation, e.g. by caries or unlined fillings

34. (a) It may become chronic, with few symptoms, either as a apical granuloma or as a radicular cyst
   (b) It may develop into an acute alveolar abscess, and in some cases discharge into the mouth

35. (a) Adjustment of light to produce good illumination
   (b) Cleaning and drying of teeth with the 3-in-1 syringe
   (c) By maintaining the probes

Physiology

Questions

General

1. What is physiology?
2. What is the smallest functional unit of an organism?
3. What are cells made of?
4. Define the following:
   (a) tissue
   (b) organs
   (c) systems
5. Why is it important that the cell membrane is permeable?
6. What is required before energy can be released in the body?
7. What is this energy for?
8. Which compound is most commonly used to produce energy?
9. What is meant by metabolism?
10. Most of the energy released in metabolism is used for what purpose?
11. State the functions of the skin
12. What are the main excretory organs of the body?
13. How is waste eliminated from the body?
14. What are the functions of the skeleton?
15. Which cells are responsible for remodelling bone?

Answers

General

1. The study of function of living organisms

2. A cell

3. Protoplasm - nucleus and cytoplasm - surrounded by a cell membrane

4. (a) Groups of cells which perform the same function
   (b) A distinct structure, composed of groups of tissues, serving a particular function
   (c) A group of organs and tissues with a common function

5. This allows small molecules of chemical substances,such as oxygen and carbon dioxide, to pass or diffuse across, usually from a higher to a lower concentration

6. Nutrients and oxygen

7. (a) Basic metabolism, just to stay alive
   (b) Activity–at the low end 'thinking', through to vigorous exercise

8. Glucose

9. The chemical change of nutritional materials
   (a) to release energy
   (b) to build or repair the tissues
   (c) the breakdown of waste ready for excretion

10. Heat to maintain body temperature

11. (a) Protection–resists mechanical damage and is a barrier against micro-organisms
    (b) Helps to maintain body temperature
    (c) Aids water balance
    (d) Sensory nerve endings provide information about the environment

12. Lungs, kidneys, gut, skin and to a lesser extent the liver

13. (a) Respiratory system removes carbon dioxide
    (b) Urinary system eliminates soluble waste plus excess water
    (c) Alimentary canal eliminates food residue, large molecule waste products and water

14. (a) To give the body shape and support
    (b) To provide attachments for muscles
    (c) To protect vital organs e.g. the brain, heart

15. (a) Osteoclasts are bone removing cells
    (b) Osteoblasts are bone forming cells

Respiration

16. Define the three types of respiration which take place in the body
17. What is the respiratory process?
18. What is the respiratory cycle and rate?
19. Give the parts of the respiratory system
20. Name, in order, the passages and tissues through which oxygen passes from the environment to a pulmonary capillary
21. What are the basic principles of all types of artificial respiration?
22. What are the common causes of rapid breathing in a healthy person?
23. In which three aspects does expired air differ from the air breathed in?
24. Give the functions of the nasal passages
25. What passes through the oropharynx?
26. How is food and fluid prevented from entering the lungs?
27. During dental treatment what are the consequences of the dropping of filling fragments to the back of the mouth?
28. How can this type of accident be prevented?

Respiration

16. (a) External–in the lungs between air and the pulmonary circulation
   (b) Internal–in the tissues between blood vessels and tissue fluid
   (c) Tissue–between tissue fluid and the cells

17. The transfer of gases, oxygen and carbon dioxide, between the environment and the body cells

18. The three phases of breathing–inspiration, expiration and brief pause. This occurs about 15 times per minute–the respiratory rate

19. (a) The airway–a series of passages along which gases can pass
   (b) The ventilation system–a nerve-controlled muscle system which helps to move the gases in the airway
   (c) The exchange area–the surface of the lungs where gases are exchanged between the air and the blood

20. Nose, nasopharynx, larynx, trachea, bronchi, bronchioles, alveolar ducts, alveoli, alveolar membrane, capillary wall, capillary

21. (a) To remove any airway obstruction
   (b) To increase and decrease the volume of the chest cavity encouraging the movement of air into and out of the lungs

22. Exercise, fear, excitement

23. Less oxygen, more carbon dioxide and water vapour

24. (a) The passage of air
   (b) Filtration–by nasal hairs
   (c) Cleansing–smaller particles and micro-organisms adhere to the mucus
   (d) Moistening–as air passes over mucus
   (e) Smell–detection of odours
   (f) Warming as air passes through

25. Air, food and fluids

26. The epiglottis guarding the entrance to the larynx is raised to the base of the tongue during swallowing so closing the airway.

27. (a) They may be swallowed
   (b) They may be inhaled. At best they may cause a bout of coughing, at worst they may enter the lungs

28. (a) Trying not to drop debris on to the tongue by care and by slight rotation of the head to one side
   (b) Efficient suction
   (c) Use of sponge packs or gauze swabs
   (d) Use of a rubber dam

29. Why is the supine position not suitable for some patients with some chest conditions?

30. Under general anaesthesia the patient's airway is at risk–why is this?

31. How can the airway be protected from debris during a general anaesthetic?

32. Why is careful removal of mouth debris important during dental treatment under sedation?

33. How can a good airway be maintained during recovery from a general anaesthetic?

29. In these diseases lung secretions reduce the efficiency of their lungs and the patients become breathless when laid flat

30. (a) The protective cough reflex is lost when the patient is anaesthetized
 (b) During operative procedures the tongue may be pushed back to obstruct the oropharynx
 (c) Depression of the mandible may obstruct the larynx

31. (a) By use of a throat pack around the endotracheal anaesthetic tube
 (b) By use of a mouth pack during a 'dental gas'
 (c) By careful working in the mouth not to disturb the pack
 (d) By thorough cleaning of the oral cavity before removal of the pack

32. The sleepy patient may be slow to swallow and a bout of coughing may upset the sedation.

33. (a) By placing the patient on his/her side in the recovery position
 (b) By extending the patient's neck by raising the chin
 (c) By keeping the mandible forward to prevent the tongue obstructing the oropharynx
 (d) Removal by suction of fluids such as blood

Nervous system

34. What is the function of the nervous system?
35. List the stimuli and name the sense organs which receive them
36. Name the parts of the nervous system
37. What is the basic unit of the nervous system?
38. Name the three types of nerve found in the body
39. State the two types of nerve response and briefly indicate how they work
40. How can messages from nerves be interrupted?

Nervous system

34. (a) The receipt and transmission of information about the body and its environment
   (b) The interpretation of that information and decision on the action necessary
   (c) The transmission of messages for action to the tissues or organs

35. (a) Light–the eyes
   (b) Smell–the nose
   (c) Sound–the ears
   (d) Pressure–the skin
   (e) Chemicals–smell (nose) and taste (tongue)
   (f) Gravity–the inner ear

36. (a) Central nervous system consisting of:
      (i) brain
      (ii) spinal cord
      (iii) cranial and peripheral nerves
   (b) Autonomic system, which controls the major systems e.g. circulation, respiration, digestion

37. The neurone

38. Sensory, motor and mixed

39. (a) Voluntary–when thought is involved.
      A stimulus is detected by peripheral neurones, the message is carried to the brain, interpreted and a response takes place e.g. a sound is heard and the head is turned towards the source
   (b) Involuntary (or reflex)–with no thought involved.
      The stimulus detected by the peripheral neurone, although passing to the brain, provokes a response as soon as it reaches the spinal cord. This is called the reflex arc and is a protective response e.g. a pinprick leads to instant withdrawal

40. By anaesthetic agents or by trauma

Heart

41. List the main parts of the circulatory system
42. Give the names of the circulatory systems
43. Using a correct order give the parts of the blood-circulating system
44. What is meant by the term 'blood pressure'?
45. What is meant by the 'pulse'?
46. What basic information can be learnt from feeling the pulse?
47. What is the function of heart valves?
48. What are the names of the chambers of the heart and what is the function of each?
49. Which type of blood is found in the pulmonary vein?
50. How do the heart muscles obtain their blood?
51. Under what circumstances might the blood pressure rise for a short period of time in a healthy person?
52. Give the normal resting heart rate for adults

Heart

41. The heart, blood vessels and lymphatic system
42. Systemic and pulmonary
43. Heart, arteries, arterioles, capillaries, venules, veins
44. It is the pressure of the flow of blood on the arterial walls
45. It is the pressure wave set up in the arterial walls when the heart pumps more blood into the arteries
46. The heart rate can be determined
47. To allow blood to flow in one direction only
48. Right atrium–collection of blood from the tissues
    Right ventricle–pumps blood via the pulmonary arteries to the lungs
    Left atrium–receives blood from the pulmonary veins
    Left ventricle–pumps blood via the aorta and arterial system to the tissues
49. Oxygenated blood
50. Via the coronary arteries
51. With strenuous exercise or with fear
52. 70 beats per minute

Blood

53. What are the two main constituents of blood and their proportions?
54. What is the volume of blood in the average adult?
55. Name the three main types of cells found in blood
56. Give the function of each type of cell
57. What are the main constituents of the fluid part of blood?
58. How is oxygen transported in the blood?
59. How is carbon dioxide transported in the blood?
60. What are the main constituents of a blood clot?
61. What is the purpose of the blood-clotting process?
62. What is the role of blood platelets in blood coagulation?
63. What part does fibrin play in blood clotting?
64. How do blood vessels help to reduce blood loss?
65. What is 'haemophilia', how is it passed on and whom does it affect?
66. What is meant by 'thrombosis' and which human organ does it frequently affect?
67. Why might thrombus formation seriously damage a person?
68. Why must the dental surgeon know if a patient is taking anticoagulant drugs?
69. What is anaemia?
70. Why might a person develop a blue colour?
71. What is 'lymph'?
72. What is the function of the lymphatic system?
73. What is the function of lymph nodes?

Blood

53. Plasma–55%; cells–45%
54. 5 litres (70 ml per kg of body weight)
55. Red cells, white cells and platelets
56. Red cells–oxygen transport
    White cells–defence
    Platelets–blood clotting
57. Water (90%), nutrients, oxygen, chemical substances e.g. waste products, hormones, enzymes
58. Attached to the haemoglobin of the red cells
59. Mainly dissolved in plasma. A small amount is attached to haemoglobin
60. Fibrin, platelets, red and white cells
61. (a) To prevent excessive blood loss
    (b) To start the repair process
    (c) To stop further entry of micro-organisms
62. When damaged they produce thromboplastin which helps to produce fibrin
63. It forms a network of fibres which trap blood cells to form the blood clot
64. Contraction of the elastic layer reduces their size
65. (a) Absence of a factor in the blood-clotting chain leading to prolonged bleeding
    (b) Genetically by female carriers
    (c) Affects males only
66. Formation of blood clots within blood vessels. The heart
67. It blocks a blood vessel and reduces the oxygen supply to that area of tissue, which in some organs may seriously affect the person especially when the brain and heart are involved
68. The blood will not clot normally due to these drugs. The treatment plan may have to be modified or the patient's doctor consulted before any surgical treatment is carried out.
69. Low haemoglobin content of blood
70. Due to poor oxygenation of the blood. The blueness is called 'cyanosis'
71. Tissue fluid within lymph vessels
72. (a) To collect tissue fluids from tissues and return them to the blood-stream
    (b) To collect excretory products from the cells
    (c) To produce certain white cells
    (d) To transport fat from the small intestine
73. (a) To filter off and destroy micro-organisms and foreign bodies
    (b) To manufacture lymphocytes

Digestion

74. Why is digestion necessary?
75. Name the four main aspects of alimentary canal activity
76. Name the major glands associated with digestion
77. What factors affect the flow of saliva?
78. What is the function of the pancreas?
79. What is the function of the liver?
80. What are the essential constituents of the diet?
81. 'The diet should be adequate and balanced'–what is meant by this statement?
82. Give the important factors which affect the amount of food required by a person
83. What are the effects of between-meals snacks?
84. Where does the first stage of digestion take place?
85. Briefly explain what happens in the first stage of digestion
86. What protective actions occur during swallowing?

Digestion

74. Complex food molecules need to be broken down into smaller, absorbable and useful molecules. Insoluble substances need to be converted into soluble sustances if possible

75. Ingestion–digestion–absorption–elimination

76. Salivary–pancreas–liver

77. Increased by:
    (a) sight and smell of food
    (b) objects in the mouth e.g. dentures
    Decreased by:
    (a) some diseases
    (b) X-radiation
    (c) some drugs
    (d) age

78. (a) To produce pancreatic juice–digestive enzymes and alkali
    (b) To secrete hormones including insulin

79. (a) To change the chemical composition of substances ready for use by the body or for storage or for excretion
    (b) Formation of bile to aid digestion
    (c) Storage of glycogen, iron and vitamins
    (d) Detoxication of drugs and toxins
    (e) Heat production to help maintain body temperature

80. Carbohydrates (starch and sugars), fats, proteins, mineral salts, water, vitamins and roughage

81. 'adequate'–enough for energy and growth needs
    'balanced'–all the essential constituents should be present in the correct proportions

82. Age, build, sex, type of activity performed e.g. occupation

83. (a) They spoil the appetite for balanced meals
    (b) Can lead to obesity as they are usually high in calories
    (c) Encourage dental disease

84. In the mouth

85. Biting and chewing of food mixes it with saliva. The saliva contains the enzyme ptyalin or amylase which starts the digestion of starches

86. (a) The nasal cavity is protected by the soft palate and the posterior pharyngeal wall
    (b) The larynx is protected by the closure of the epiglottis

87. What is the action of the tongue in mastication?

88. What is the purpose of the masticatory process?

89. What is meant by a digestive enzyme?

90. How long may the gastric digestive process take?

91. Why does the alimentary canal secrete mucous?

92. Why is gastric juice acid?

93. Give two examples of foods which are absorbed through the stomach walls into the bloodstream

94. What part of the digestive process takes place
    (a) in the ileum
    (b) in the colon

95. Why are nasal and oral secretions necessary to perceive the senses of smell and taste?

96. Where are the majority of taste buds found?

97. What are the basic taste sensations and where are they detected?

87. (a) To help to mix food particles with saliva
   (b) To help to keep food between the teeth

88. (a) To produce a large surface area for the action of enzymes
   (b) To produce pieces of food of a reasonable size for swallowing

89. An organic catalyst which speeds the rate of chemical breakdown of food

90. Frequently as long as three hours, sometimes even longer hence the period of 'nil by mouth' prior to a general anaesthetic

91. To lubricate the food and to protect the walls of the alimentary canal

92. (a) To kill micro-organisms
   (b) Gastric enzymes need an acid medium
   (c) To stop the action of amylase

93. Simple molecule foods, e.g. glucose, alcohol

94. (a) Absorption of end-products of digestion
   (b) Water absorption

95. These are chemical senses and therefore need the odour or flavour to be in solution to stimulate the sensory nerve endings. It is a protective mechanism against poisoning

96. On the upper (dorsal) surface of the tongue

97. (a) Sweet and salt, mainly at the tip of the tongue
   (b) Sour, at the sides of the tongue
   (c) Bitter, at the back of the tongue

General disease

Questions

1. Define the following words:
   (a) disease
   (b) aetiology
   (c) idiopathic
   (d) pathology
   (e) congenital

2. What is the term applied to the defence reaction of the body to injury or irritation?

3. What is the difference between the symptoms and the signs of disease?

4. Define the following words:
   (a) syndrome
   (b) fever

5. How may infection spread in the body?

6. What is an abscess and what are its contents?

7. Name the two types of inflammation. How do they differ?

8. What are the objectives of the inflammatory reaction?

9. List the factors which affect healing.

10. What are the results of acute inflammation?

11. What are the results of chronic inflammation?

12. What is an ulcer?

13. What is meant by the term 'healing by first intention'?

14. What is meant by 'healing by secondary intention'?

Answers

1. (a) Departure from normal anatomy, physiology and biochemistry
   (b) The study of factors which cause disease
   (c) Of unknown cause
   (d) The study of disease and the factors which cause disease
   (e) Present from birth
2. Inflammation
3. Patients complain of their symptoms; doctors and dentists detect signs.
4. (a) A set of signs and symptoms which occur in a fixed pattern
   (b) Increased body temperature due to disease
5. By blood system, lymphatic system or by spread through adjacent tissues
6. A collection of pus contained within a cavity lined by a pyogenic membrane. It contains inflammatory exudate, tissue debris, white cells and micro-organisms.
7. (a) Acute–usually lasting hours or days
   (b) Chronic–lasting weeks or months
      In the acute form the cause is too severe for the local body defences to overcome and the total body defences are called into action. In the chronic form the cause is much less severe and there is a slow smouldering reaction in which repair and destruction occur simultaneously
8. (a) To destroy or remove the cause or the by-products
   (b) To limit damage to the body
   (c) To repair or replace damaged tissues
9. (a) General–health, age, nutrition etc.
   (b) Local
      (i) Open or closed wound
      (ii) Blood supply, a poor supply retards healing
      (iii) Infection may be the cause or may develop at the site
      (iv) Foreign body retained e.g. splinter
      (v) Further injury
10. (a) Resolution and repair
    (b) Cause not completely overcome leading to partial resolution and to chronic inflammation
11. A 'walling-off' type of reaction which may restrict the blood supply to the area and delay complete healing
12. A persistent break in a body surface
13. Where the edges of a wound stick together and join e.g. a stab-type cut
14. Where there is a gap in the wound which has to be bridged e.g. loss of a deep area of skin. Healing takes place from the edges and the base and is a much slower process

Medical conditions

15. What is a haemorrhage?
16. What is the physiological arrest of haemorrhage called?
17. What is meant by 'anaemia'?
18. What is a haemophiliac?
19. Treating a haemophiliac carries with it certain risks; what are they?
20. What is a thrombus?
21. What damage can a thrombus cause?
22. What is meant by the term 'a stroke'?
23. What is angina pectoris?
24. What is meant by coronary thrombosis?
25. Why are some patients with cardiovascular disease sometimes prescribed anticoagulant drugs by their doctors?
26. For a patients with cardiovascular disease, how might his/her dental treatment be affected?
27. What is meant by congenital heart disease?
28. Why are antibiotics given before some dental procedures to patients with a history of rheumatic fever, heart valve disease etc?

Medical conditions

15. The abnormal loss of blood from a blood vessel

16. Blood clotting

17. Lack of haemoglobin. This leads to a lack of oxygen carrying capacity of blood resulting in symptoms such as tiredness, pallor etc.

18. A male with an hereditary bleeding disorder

19. (a) Persistent bleeding if the soft tissues are damaged
    (b) Transmission of hepatitis B or human immuno-deficiency viruses since these patients may have been given infected blood products

20. An abnormal blood clot occurring within a blood vessel

21. Fragments of a thrombus can become detached–they are known as emboli. They circulate in the bloodstream and can block small blood vessels leading to thrombosis. This will be serious if the heart, brain or lungs are affected

22. Strictly, interference in the blood supply to a part of the brain, usually caused by a blood clot or haemorrhage. Oxygen lack leads to nerve cell damage and some loss of function of the relative part of the body.

23. Usually referred to as angina. It is a severe pain in the centre of the chest due to lack of oxygen in the heart muscle, brought on by anxiety and exertion.

24. A 'heart attack'. When a blood clot blocks the blood supply to an area of heart muscle.

25. To reduce the danger of blood clots forming in damaged blood vessels

26. General anaesthesia is usually contraindicated, also local anaesthetic solutions containing adrenaline. If anticoagulant drugs are being taken the doctor may need to adjust the dosage to prevent excessive haemorrhage

27. Abnormal development of part of the heart. This is often corrected by surgery and the patient lives a normal life.

28. During treatment additional micro-organisms may get into the bloodstream and might cause further damage in an already damaged heart

29. What is meant by infective endocarditis?

30. What is bronchitis?

31. What are the common causes of bronchitis?

32. List the signs of chronic bronchitis which a DA might notice.

33. What is asthma?

34. What is diabetes?

35. How is diabetes in a patient important to the dental surgeon?

36. Why are dental patients asked if they have suffered from jaundice?

37. Why is the dental surgeon interested to know if a patient suffers from rheumatoid arthritis?

38. What is meant by epilepsy?

39. Why is it important that the correct record cards are available before the patient enters the surgery?

40. What can the receptionist do to help the medically sick patient?

29. Inflammation of the lining of the heart. Patients may become seriously ill needing long hospitalization. It can be prevented by giving prophylactic antibiotics.

30. Inflammation of the bronchial tubes

31. Air pollution, cigarette smoking, repeated attacks of acute bronchitis, chronic infection of the nasal sinuses

32. Chronic cough and sputum, worse in the mornings
Breathlessness on exertion, due to poor oxygen uptake in the lungs

33. Difficult breathing due to spasm of the muscles of the bronchi. Attacks usually last a few minutes and known sufferers carry an aerosol inhaler.

34. There are two forms but it usually means a condition where there is a lack of insulin, so that there is low absorption of glucose.

35. (a) Under the stress of dentistry a diabetic patient may get out of sugar balance and develop a diabetic crisis. The safest action is giving sugar but urgent medical care is essential.
    (b) These patients have a low resistance to infection so that a poor gingival and periodontal condition is common, as are dry sockets.

36. Jaundice is a yellow discoloration of the skin and may be due to liver damage which could, in turn, be due to hepatitis B

37. Some of these patients are prescribed steroid drugs over many years and they become less able to cope with surgical stress and may collapse. They are also prone to infection. The arthritis may cause mobility problems e.g. getting into a dental chair and in cleaning the mouth

38. A disorder of brain activity characterized by fits usually of unknown cause

39. (a) To give the operator time to check the medical notes, among other things
    (b) If necessary to take steps to prevent medical and dental problems arising

40. Try to arrange appointments at a time most suitable to the patient and the operator, in order to ensure the greatest patient co-operation and comfort

First aid

Questions

1. What is meant by first aid?
2. Why should a DA know some first aid?
3. Before attending to the victim what should the helper consider?
4. What are the objectives of first aid?
5. What patient needs should be assessed?
6. How can the first aider find the possible cause of the problem?
7. To monitor a patient what should the DA observe and how?
8. Why is it important for the dental surgeon to get a full medical history, and to know of any drugs which the patient is taking?
9. How can a DA help to prevent injury to a conscious patient during dental treatment?
10. List some common causes of collapse
11. What action should be taken when a person collapses?

Answers

1. Skilled immediate care in the case of injury or illness. This care should continue until the person recovers or more skilled help takes over

2. (a) To be able to assist someone in need wherever they are
   (b) In particular, to assist at any emergency at the workplace

3. (a) Briefly find out what has happened
   (b) Attend to external causes e.g. cut off gas, electricity etc

4. (a) Preserve life
   (b) Prevent deterioration of the victim
   (c) Promote recovery

5. (a) Check breathing
   (b) Check for bleeding
   (c) Check state of consciousness
   (d) Decide how best to assist and call for other help

6. (a) Ask victim and witnesses what happened
   (b) Note victim's symptoms
   (c) Elicit signs using sight, hearing, smell and touch
   Remember you are not asked to diagnose but you need to know about the cause in order to help

7. (a) Colour of lips, forehead etc, whether pale, flushed or blue
   (b) Skin, whether clammy or dry
   (c) Chest–rate and amount of rise and fall
   (d) That air passes through nose or mouth
   (e) Pulse–if there is one and then what is the rate

8. (a) To prevent adverse reactions or emergencies
   (b) To plan treatment taking into account the medical history
   (c) To carry out treatment knowing the possible problems which might occur

9. (a) Careful suction and guarding of the cheeks and tongue
   (b) By asking the patient to wear protective goggles
   (c) By making sure instruments are cool
   (d) By not passing instruments or materials across the patient's face

10. Fainting, shock, asphyxia, diabetes, epilepsy, associated with heart and kidney diseases, poisoning

11. (a) Ensure that the patient can breathe properly
    (b) Try to decide cause of collapse
    (c) Carry out appropriate simple treatment e.g. try to stop bleeding
    (d) Summon help as soon as possible
    In the surgery dental procedures naturally would cease immediately

12. Into what position should an unconscious person be placed and why?

13. Certain types of person should not be put into this position–who are they and why?

14. How can the dental team ensure that a patient gets plenty of oxygen?

15. When a person loses consciousness why is it important to ensure a good oxygen intake?

16. Give the normal rate of respiration

17. What is meant by asphyxia?

18. What are the signs and symptoms of asphyxia?

19. Give the causes of asphyxia

20. What is the objective in giving artificial respiration?

21. In mouth-to-mouth resuscitation, how can one assess that the lungs are being inflated?

22. For how long is resuscitation continued?

23. Why should no drink or food be given to an unconscious person?

24. What are the signs and symptoms of fainting?

25. A person who faints naturally falls to the ground; how does this aid recovery?

26. What is shock?

27. What are the symptoms of shock?

12. The tonsillar or recovery position. This enables the person to breathe freely and fluids to drain out of the mouth

13. Anyone with a suspected spinal injury; however, a good airway must be maintained to prevent brain damage

14. (a) Secure the airway:
    (i) Check that there is no obstruction in the mouth, pharynx or larynx
    (ii) Check that there is no restriction to breathing e.g. tight clothing
    (b) After these checks administer oxygen

15. Deprivation of oxygen can lead to severe brain damage

16. 15 times per minute

17. Lack of oxygen in the tissues, in particular the brain

18. (a) Obvious difficulty in breathing
    (b) Blueness of extremities (called cyanosis)
    (c) Confusion, leading to unconsciousness, leading to cardiac arrest

19. (a) Lack of oxygen in the air e.g. gas, smoke
    (b) Airway obstruction
    (i) external e.g. pillow, plastic bag
    (ii) internal: anatomical e.g. tongue; foreign body e.g. vomit, sea water
    (c) Damage to the nervous system e.g. poisoning, electrocution

20. To maintain supply of some oxygen to the blood and so to the tissues.

21. By observing the rise and fall of the chest, not of the abdomen

22. For as long as necessary or until a doctor pronounces the person dead

23. (a) They might inhale the food or drink directly or during regurgitation if they vomit

    (b) A general anaesthetic might have to be delayed because of the intake of food or fluid

24. The patient appears distressed, pale, sweaty and yet cold, dizzy and nauseated and may lose consciousness briefly. The pulse is rapid and weak

25. Because of the position there will be increased venous blood to the heart: therefore some cardiac output will be maintained and the heart will more easily pump some blood to the brain

26. Sudden and severe drop in blood pressure

27. Nausea, vomiting, fainting

28. What are the signs of shock?
29. What are the causes of shock?
30. How would you treat a person with shock?
31. What are the consequences of severe haemorrhage?
32. What is the first aid treatment of cardiac arrest?
33. What is the first aid treatment of non-dental haemorrhage?
34. A patient collapses on the floor and is having convulsions. What might be the reasons for these convulsions?
35. Give the signs of an epileptic fit–grand mal
36. How should you help a person having an epileptic fit?
37. What is the difference between a burn and a scald?
38. What is the first aid treatment of burns?
39. Give the first aid treatment in cases of electrocution
40. Why might a pregnant woman faint even in the supine position?
41. What first aid treatment would you give to a person with a suspected fractured bone?

28. Pallor, sweating, pulse rapid and weak, consciousness at a lowered level and may even become unconscious, staying so until medical treatment is given

29. Primary shock–fear, pain, alarm, temper
Secondary shock–prolonged or severe loss of blood

30. (a) Lay them down and keep warm but not overheated
(b) Untreated secondary shock can lead to permanent damage and death, so it is important to summon medical help urgently
(c) If person is bleeding try to stop the haemorrhage
(d) Get help

31. Loss of blood pressure, of red cells, of oxygen, cardiac arrest, death

32. Chest compression (formerly known as external cardiac massage), i.e. apply pressure to the sternum about 60 times per minute

33. (a) Apply pressure to the wound to stop the bleeding
(b) Elevate the part, which helps to reduce blood flow
(c) Get the patient to rest
(d) Summon help

34. Epilepsy, hysteria. There are other less common reasons

35. Patients have a warning–an aura. Loss of consciousness sometimes with alternate muscle contraction and relaxation. Incontinence

36. (a) Prevent injury by removing obvious danger e.g. electric fire
(b) Do not restrain but when fit subsides ensure airway
(c) After a fit the person often falls asleep–let them wake naturally
(d) If fit continues or a second one occurs call for medical help
(e) In any case after recovery person must be accompanied home
Contrary to belief the tongue is rarely bitten, more likely the first aider's fingers. Inserting a hard object between the teeth tends to damage the teeth e.g. breaking cusps or incisal corners

37. A burn is caused by dry heat, a scald by wet heat

38. (a) Remove the cause
(b) Cool the area with water
(c) Prevent or treat shock
(d) Cover with a sterile dressing which has been wetted with sterile cold water or cover with clean plastic film

39. (a) Switch off the electricity supply
(b) Apply artificial respiration if necessary
(c) Treat as for burns

40. The foetus may press on the inferior vena cava and restrict the return of blood to the heart

41. (a) If possible immobilize the part
(b) Get person to hospital–probably by ambulance

Drugs

Questions

1. In medicine, what is a drug?
2. What is meant by drug abuse?
3. Define, in relation to drugs, the following terms:
   (a) tolerance
   (b) dependence
   (c) addiction
4. How are drugs admnistered medically?
5. What is meant by the side-effects of drugs?
6. What is the use of the following drugs:
   (a) aralgesics
   (b) hypnotics
   (c) tranquillizers
   (d) sedatives
7. What are antimicrobial drugs?
8. Briefly define the following:
   (a) disinfectants
   (b) antiseptics

Answers

1. A substance taken to aid recovery from sickness or to relieve symptoms, or to modify a natural process in the body

2. (a) Persistent taking of medicines which are not needed medically. This has wide implications and, for example, includes excessive use of laxatives
   (b) The taking of drugs which are not socially acceptable

3. (a) Becoming used to a drug so that increasing amounts are required to produce the same effect; this can apply to common drugs such as aspirin
   (b) Physical and mental craving for pleasure or relief of discomfort
   (c) Four characteristics–craving, tolerance, dependence and harmful effects on the person

4. (a) Through the skin or mucous membrane
   (b) Via body orifices–orally, rectally
   (c) Into muscles–intramuscular
   (d) Into veins–intravenous

5. (a) Most drugs cause some unwanted, but acceptable, effects on the body e.g. kill non-pathogenic microbes, sometimes this may be a problem such as gastric upsets with antibiotics
   (b) Some drugs, when mixed with others, produce exaggerated effects e.g. alcohol taken during a course of metronidazole
   (c) Some drugs affect the developing child, leading to abnormalities e.g. tetracycline on forming enamel; thalidomide on forming limbs

6. (a) For relief of pain
   (b) To induce sleep
   (c) To calm and promote a feeling of well-being, to reduce anxiety
   (d) To soothe or make drowsy

7. Chemical agents which interfere with the growth and multiplication of all types of micro-organisms

8. (a) Powerful chemical agents which destroy many living organisms as well as living tissue. Now called 'environmental disinfectants'
   (b) Chemical agents, sometimes diluted disinfectants, which inhibit the growth of microbes and are usually less harmful to tissues. Now called 'surface disinfectants'

9. How should drugs be stored?

10. How should unwanted unscheduled drugs (not dangerous) be disposed of?

11. List the types of drugs commonly kept in dental surgeries

12. Drugs are sometimes given to prevent disease. What is the term used to describe this type of therapy?

13. What advice should be given to a patient about taking pain-killing drugs following dental treatment?

14. When can the DA give analgesics to a patient?

15. What are the differences between an antiseptic and an antibiotic?

16. Antibiotics are said to have a 'spectrum' of action; what does this mean?

17. What special property does metronidazole (Flagyl) have so that it is prescribed for gum infections?

18. What is meant by 'penicillin sensitivity'?

9. (a) In a cool dry place out of reach of children and preferably locked
   (b) All containers should be clearly labelled including expiry date
   (c) Containers must have well-fitting tops, preferably 'child proof'
   (d) All drugs should be used in date order
   (e) Drugs on which people may be dependent, e.g. analgesics, tranquillizers, must be kept in a locked cupboard. Prescription pads should be kept in a secure place

10. (a) By mixing with water and pouring down a drain, or
   (b) By returning them to a pharmacy. Under no circumstances should they be thrown in a waste bin as they could then be 'found' and taken

11. (a) Anaesthetic agents–local and general including intravenous drugs
   (b) Sedation drugs
   (c) Emergency resuscitation drugs
   (d) Analgesics

12. Prophylactic drug therapy

13. As a general rule the DA should not advise on drugs, but common sense advice to patients would be for them to take the usual dose of the pain killer they normally take. Advising other analgesics could be dangerous.

14. Analgesics should only be given out on the written instructions of and checked by a dental surgeon. An entry on the patient's record card is sufficient and should be endorsed 'Given' plus the initials of the DA

15. (a) Antiseptic–a chemical which prevents the growth of bacteria (bacteriostasis) and which may kill some bacteria (bacteriocidal)
   (b) Antibiotic–a biological substance which kills or inhibits the growth of certain micro-organisms. Some antibiotics can be produced synthetically

16. Each antibiotic is effective in killing certain types of micro-organisms only–this is the spectrum. Most of the pathogens related to dentistry are killed by penicillin but in hospital dental practice a wider range of micro-organisms has to be dealt with

17. It is mainly effective against anaerobic organisms and these proliferate in deep periodontal pockets

18. An adverse reaction of the body to penicillin. At its simplest the development of a body rash; at its most dangerous, collapse and death

19. Why is it important that patients should complete the course of antibiotics?

20. What problems can arise with penicillin therapy?

21. In which medical conditions might penicillin be given prophylactically before dental treatment?

22. Why is prophylactic penicillin prescribed for these patients?

23. What is a fungicide? Give an example of a fungicide used in dentistry.

24. Why might a patient be taking anticoagulant drugs?

25. What is a drug warning card?

26. Why is premedication sometimes given to a patient?

27. How is premedication administered in dentistry? Name a drug commonly used

28. Why might a patient be taking steroid drugs?

29. What is the effect of steroid drugs on the body?

30. What are the basic principles in the treatment of poisoning?

19. (a) To bring the infection under control of the body's defences
(b) To prevent the development of resistant strains of micro-organisms

20. (a) The patient may be allergic to the drug
(b) Sometimes gastro-intestinal upsets occur

21. Where there is a history of rheumatic heart disease, heart valve disorder, heart murmurs, if the patient has undergone open heart surgery or major organ transplant

22. During treatment, oral micro-organisms may enter the blood-stream, settle on the damaged tissues, multiply and lead to a serious medical condition known as infective endocarditis

23. A substance which kills fungi. Nystatin or Amphotericin B used in the treatment of denture sore mouth which is caused by a fungus (*Candida albicans*)

24. To reduce the risk of blood clotting in vessels. Usually associated with cardiovascular disease

25. A card issued by doctors to patients taking medicines which alter their normal reaction to injury or stress e.g. anticoagulants, steroid drugs

26. (a) To allay fear
(b) To make the patient more co-operative
(c) To help produce a smooth general anaesthetic
(d) To reduce secretions e.g. salivary flow

27. Usually orally. Diazepam

28. In the treatment of medical conditions such as rheumatoid arthritis, asthma and some skin diseases

29. They suppress inflammatory response. An unwanted side-effect is to reduce the natural production of cortico-steroids. This will reduce patients' ability to withstand stress, and they are more likely to collapse

30. (a) Identify the poison if possible
(b) Give specific or general antidote if the poison is corrosive
(c) If the poison is non-corrosive, encourage vomiting
(d) Get medical assistance

Local anaesthesia

Questions

1. What is meant by the words:
   (a) anaesthesia
   (b) analgesia
   (c) paraesthesia

2. What factors influence a patient's ability to describe pain?

3. Name the parts of the central nervous system.

4. How are painful stimuli detected by the body?

5. What is the body's immediate reaction to a painful stimulus?

6. Which cranial nerve is involved with the jaws and teeth?

7. Which types of nerve fibres does it contain?

8. Which branches of this cranial nerve supply the upper and lower teeth?

9. Give the uses of local analgesia in dentistry

10. What are the advantages of local analgesia for most dental procedures?

11. What are the disadvantages of local anaesthesia?

12. Apart from local and general anaesthesia what other techniques are available to help patients to accept dental treatment?

13. In which four basic ways can local analgesia be obtained?

Answers

1. (a) Loss of all sensation
   (b) Loss of pain sensation
   (c) Altered sensation, i.e. a tingling feeling in the area supplied by that nerve

2. Most important is the ability to express feelings in words. This ability is influenced by age, education, previous experience etc.

3. (a) The brain and cranial nerves
   (b) The spinal cord and spinal nerves

4. By sensory neurones

5. The reflex protective one of moving away. However a conscious decision can be taken to over-ride this reaction e.g. the benefits of an injection outweigh the painful prick sensation

6. The fifth or trigeminal

7. Sensory and motor

8. Upper–superior dental branches of the maxillary nerve
   Lower–inferior dental branch of the mandibular nerve

9. (a) Elimination of pain during operative procedures
   (b) As an aid to diagnosis of facial pain

10. (a) Safe–side-effects and complications uncommon; minimum aftercare e.g. patient can drive
    (b) Medical state–can be administered to most patients if suitable precautions are taken
    (c) Time–virtually unlimited operating time
    (d) Patient co-operation for all procedures

11. (a) Needle injection required for full analgesia
    (b) Does not work effectively in the presence of inflammation or pus
    (c) Patient discomfort from loss of sensation
    (d) Patient needs to be careful not to damage numb area

12. (a) A good relationship between the patient and the operator and DA
    (b) What is usually described as 'tender loving care'
    (c) Various forms of sedation–oral, inhalation or intravenous

13. (a) Local infiltration
    (b) Regional or block technique
    (c) Intra-ligamentary
    (d) Surface application (topical)

14. How does a local anaesthetic drug work?
15. Why is local analgesia seldom used where there is an abscess?
16. In what forms are surface anaesthetics supplied?
17. What are the uses of a surface anaesthetic?
18. List the contents of any local anaesthetic cartridge
19. At what temperature should the cartridge be used and why?
20. Why are cartridges packed in 'bubble packs'?
21. How can the needle diaphragm of a cartridge be disinfected?
22. What are the advantages of disposable needles for local anaesthesia?
23. What types of disposable needle are there?
24. What is an intra-ligamentary injection anaesthetic?
25. When is the 'short' needle fitted to the syringe?
26. What should the DA check before loading a local anaesthetic cartridge into the syringe?

14. It blocks nerve impulses along the sensory pathway

15. (a) The infection may be spread by the procedure
    (b) Local analgesics are less efficient in the presence of inflammation due to the acidity of the tissues

16. Ointment, solution, spray and lozenges

17. (a) Analgesia of the mucous membrane or skin to aid painless insertion of a syringe needle
    (b) An aid to the removal of very loose deciduous teeth
    (c) Analgesia to allow incision of an abscess
    (d) For minor procedures involving the gingiva
    (e) In some cases for deep scaling

18. (a) Anaesthetic agent
    (b) Usually a vasoconstrictor
    (c) An antiseptic
    (d) A preservative
    (e) Isotonic water for injection

19. 30–40 °C i.e. about body temperature; outside these limits there is pain on injection of the solution

20. This is a sterile pack and, in particular, the cap where the needle is inserted is sterile

21. Care should be taken to remove the cartridge from the bubble pack only when it is needed and loaded into the syringe. Should a minor contamination occur then the diaphragm can either be dipped in fresh antiseptic solution or flamed

22. (a) They are always sharp
    (b) They are very thin, therefore easier penetration is obtained
    (c) They are already sterile
    (d) There is reduced risk of transmitting infection, particularly hepatitis B

23. (a) Cartridge–long or short, usually gauge 27 or 30; ultra-fine for intra-ligamentary
    (b) Hypodermic–various lengths, gauges 1 to 27

24. A method of producing local analgesia by injecting solution through a very fine needle into the periodontal ligament. It limits the area of anaesthesia and is short-acting

25. For infiltration anaesthetics

26. (a) The contents–anaesthetic drug and whether vasoconstrictor or not
    (b) Date of expiry

27. What would be checked after loading the syringe?

28. Why should patients be offered a mouthwash immediately after receiving a local anaesthetic injection?

29. Local anaesthetic solution placed beside lower molar teeth does not give adequate analgesia for most dental procedures–why is this?

30. Which nerves are affected by a mandibular nerve block?

31. Basically how does a mandibular nerve block work?

32. Patients may say that their lips feel swollen after receiving a mandibular nerve block–why is this?

33. What is the advantage of the aspirating syringe for the administration of local anaesthetic solutions?

34. Why do local anasthetics contain a vasoconstrictor?

35. What might be the consequences of injecting local anaesthetic solution into a blood vessel?

36. When an infiltration injection is being given the gingiva may become white–why is this?

37. What causes the local anaesthetic to wear off?

38. What is the most common complication associated with the giving of local anaesthetics, and what is the usual cause?

39. What are the signs and symptoms of the complication?

27. (a) If an aspirating syringe, that the rubber bung withdraws
 (b) That the solution flows through the needle
 (c) That any air has been expelled from the cartridge
 (d) That the cartridge details can be read and checked by the operator

28. The taste is very bitter

29. The solution has difficulty in penetrating the dense alveolar bone in this area

30. The inferior dental and lingual nerves, sometimes the long buccal as well

31. Anaesthetic solution is placed beside the nerve before it enters the mandible through the mandibular foramen. The nerve is anaesthetized at this point, preventing impulses passing back to the brain

32. The mental nerve which is sensory to the lower lip is a terminal branch of the mandibular nerve. With the loss of sensation the lip feels thick but in fact no change has taken place

33. It allows the operator to check that the injection is not about to be given into a blood vessel

34. (a) To restrict diffusion of the local anaesthetic solution which will
  (i) prolong the period of analgesia
  (ii) ensure a high level of analgesia
 (b) The haemostatic effect is sometimes useful in surgery

35. It may cause the patient to faint. The heart rate may rise and the patient may complain of being aware of his/her heart beating

36. (a) Pressure within the tissues from the volume of solution
 (b) The vasoconstrictor affecting the small vessels at the site injection

37. The concentration of the solution declines as it is removed by tissue fluid and passes into the bloodstream

38. Fainting, due to nervousness

39. Sweaty brow, pallor, nausea, patient complains of feeling unwell and hot, momentary loss of consciousness may occur

40. How can this complication be treated?

41. Why should a partly used cartridge not be used on another patient?

42. Blood is removed from forceps which are then sterilized–why are syringe needles not resterilized?

43. How can a cartridge become contaminated when an injection is given?

44. If a patient telephoned the practice a day after a 'local' stating that he/she was still numb, what would you do?

40. (a) Prevention
  (i) Patients should be encouraged to have some food or a drink beforehand to raise the blood sugar level
  (ii) Check on arrival and if necessary provide a drink
  (iii) Supine position reduces the chance of fainting

  (b) Treatment
  (i) If not already so, place patient in supine position with head as lowest point of the body; raising the legs also helps
  (ii) As patient recovers have a sweetened drink available
  (iii) Slowly raise patient to avoid a repeat faint

41. The cartridge could be contaminated and lead to cross-infection

42. It is impossible to be sure that the inside of the needle is sterile

43. As soon as injecting ceases the rubber plunger relaxes creating a negative pressure in the cartridge: as a result some tissue fluid may be sucked back into the cartridge

44. Arrange for the patient to see the operator as soon as possible. Numbness for this length of time suggests something unusual

General anaesthesia

Questions

1. What is meant by the following:
   (a) anaesthesia
   (b) analgesia
   (c) anaesthetics

2. How is general anaesthesia produced?

3. What are the indications for giving a dental general anaesthetic?

4. Give the main reason why general anaesthesia is avoided in pregnancy?

5. Which drugs are commonly administered for dental general anaesthesia by:
   (a) inhalation
   (b) injection

6. How long does it take for an intravenous (i.v.) drug to travel from the arm to the brain?

7. Some anaesthetists give an injection to get the patient 'to sleep' and then continue with anaesthetic gases. Why is this technique used?

8. Why should the drugs in the emergency kit be checked regularly?

9. Why should the name of the patient's current medical practitioner be written on the patient's record card?

10. How often should the patient's medical history and drug record be checked?

11. How can a patient's fears of dentistry be allayed?

12. Why does the anaesthetist need to know the patient's weight?

13. Why should the patient be accompanied by a DA throughout a general anaesthetic?

14. What is endotracheal anaesthesia?

15. What are the most important advantages of endotracheal anaesthesia?

16. Why might the patient complain of a sore throat after an endotracheal anaesthetic?

17. Why should the patient's eyes be protected during a general anaesthetic?

Answers

1. (a) Loss of sensation in the whole body (general) or in part (local)
   (b) Loss of pain sensation only
   (c) Drugs (agents) which abolish sensation either generally or locally

2. By means of drugs administered by injection or inhalation

3. (a) Acute inflammation and the presence of pus
   (b) Multiple extractions and major surgery
   (c) Children—most probably extraction of abscessed teeth
   (d) Mentally and physically handicapped patients
   (e) Very nervous patients

4. To avoid possible damage to the foetus from the anaesthetic drugs or from hypoxia

5. (a) Nitrous oxide, halothane, enflurane, oxygen
   (b) Methohexitone, thiopentone

6. 15–20 seconds

7. (a) The patient is quickly anaesthetized which is more pleasant for the patient
   (b) The gases produce good safe analgesia with rapid recovery

8. (a) To ensure that they are all present
   (b) To check that they are not out of date

9. In case it is necessary to make contact in an emergency

10. At each examination and before prescribing or administering drugs

11. (a) By efficient pain reduced dentistry
    (b) By use of sedation, premedication or hypnosis to reduce anxiety

12. The dosage of drugs is calculated on the patient's weight among other factors e.g. age, medical state etc.

13. To act as chaperone

14. The administration of anaesthetic gases via a tube which passes through the nose and larynx into the trachea

15. (a) It secures the patient's airway
    (b) It prevents foreign substances e.g. blood, getting into the lungs
    (c) It allows better access to the mouth

16. The throat pack absorbs secretions so that there is a lack of normal lubrication

17. As the eyelid reflexes are abolished under anaesthesia it is necessary to protect them from injury e.g. corneal abrasion or infection

18. What is the oxygen content of air?

19. How do gaseous anaesthetics get to the brain?

20. What are the advantages and disadvantages of administering general anaesthetics via an intravenous route?

21. What is the usual minimum percentage of oxygen administered with nitrous oxide and why is it necessary?

22. What does the word 'hypoxia' mean?

23. How can severe hypoxia be detected?

24. Which organ is placed under stress if less than atmospheric oxygen is available?

25. What are the characteristics of nitrous oxide?

26. How is halothane administered?

27. Why is halothane used with nitrous oxide and oxygen?

28. What are the hazards in the use of halothane:
    (a) to the patient
    (b) to the dental team?

29. How is methohexitone administered?

30. What are the duties of a DA when receiving a patient who is about to have a general anaesthetic?

31. How can a DA reassure the patient before a general anaesthetic?

18. About 20%

19. The vapours diffuse from the alveoli of the lungs into the blood as it passes through the pulmonary vessels. This blood is then pumped to the brain

20. Advantages–accuracy of dosage, speed of onset, no smell, no mask
Disadvantages–some patients fear injections; great care is required in the calculation of drug dosage

21. 30%. This is necessary to maintain the blood oxygen at approximately normal level. This should ensure adequate oxygen to the brain

22. Low oxygen, i.e. less than atmospheric air

23. The patient has a bluish colour to the skin, and in severe cases there may be convulsions. The patient breathes hard in an effort to obtain sufficient oxygen

24. The heart

25. It is a colourless, non-flammable gas, with a faint smell and taste; it is supplied in cylinders. It is a weak hypnotic (sleep-inducing) drug but is used for its analgesic properties

26. It is an inhalation anaesthetic. The N_2O/O_2 gas mixture picks up halothane vapour as it passes through the halothane vaporizer

27. It produces sleep and allows at least 20% oxygen to be used while maintaining a smooth anaesthetic

28. (a) Possible liver damage if used more than once in a month
(b) Liver damage, spontaneous abortion

29. By intravenous injection. It is supplied as a white powder in a sealed bottle and is mixed with sterile water for injection to produce a 1% solution. As the law stands, the DA may carry out this duty only under the direct personal supervision of a doctor or dentist

30. (a) Confirm person's name
(b) Check that the patient has followed the pre-operation instructions, especially nil by mouth
(c) Check that the patient has no cough or cold
(d) Check that the patient has an escort home afterwards and will not drive that day
(e) Ask the patient to go to the toilet
(f) Check that the patient is wearing suitable loose clothing
(g) Check that the patient has signed the consent form
(h) Ask the patient to remove dentures and glasses, if any

31. (a) By doing her best to see that the patient is seen on time
(b) By being sympathetic with voice and actions
(c) By explaining in suitable language what will happen

32. Why should patients be asked not to eat or drink for at least 4 hours before a general anaesthetic?

33. What could be the results of vomiting under general anaesthesia?

34. Why are patients asked to wear loose clothing for an anaesthetic appointment?

35. What is the effect of a foreign body touching the vocal cords?

37. Why are throat packs used during general anaesthesia?

38. Why is it important that only the anaesthetist talks except when the patient is anaesthetised?

39. Why is it advised that dental general anaesthetics are given with the patient in the supine position?

40. How should a patient recovering from a general anaesthetic be 'monitored'?

41. Into which position should a patient be placed during recovery from a general anaesthetic?

42. Patients may 'shiver' during recovery from a general anaesthetic; why is this and how should they be cared for?

43. What are the commonest causes of collapse associated with dental general anaesthesia? Place in order of frequency of occurrence

44. Why should patients not use machinery for at least 12 hours after a general anaesthetic or intravenous sedation?

45. If a patient asks about taking pain-killing drugs after a general anaesthetic, what advice should you give?

32. (a) This gives time for the stomach to empty, which reduces the possibility of vomiting
   (b) Most fluids have time to be excreted so that a visit to the toilet before the anaesthetic should avoid incontinence

33. The laryngeal reflex is depressed during a general anaesthetic and vomit could enter the lungs, causing bronchospasm, respiratory obstruction, pneumonia or death

34. (a) Tight-fitting sleeves impede the flow of the intravenous drug to the brain
   (b) Respiration may be restricted by tight fitting clothes at the neck, chest or abdomen
   (c) In an emergency situation tight clothes may slow resuscitation

35. The cords will close to protect the lungs and prevent oxygen from reaching the lungs

36. The vocal cords are nearly closed (laryngospasm) and air passing through this restriction causes the crowing noise (called laryngeal stridor)

37. To prevent foreign bodies or saliva entering the larynx

38. The sense of hearing is the last sense to be lost and the first to return

39. It reduces the possibility of fainting. The effect of vasodilatation is reduced; thus blood pressure is less likely to fall to a level which reduces oxygenation to the brain

40. The carotid artery in the neck will usually provide a visible and palpable pulse. The chest movements can be observed, or a hand near the nose will feel the air flow

41. Into the recovery position. This is preferable to the supine position as it helps to prevent airway obstruction by the tongue and, if the patient does vomit, there is a reduced chance of inhaling the vomit

42. This may be a symptom of feeling cold or of low oxygen. Cover with a blanket; if appropriate, administer oxygen and call the anaesthetist or dental surgeon back to the recovery area

43. (a) Respiratory obstruction
   (b) Hypotension (low blood pressure)
   (c) Respiratory arrest
   (d) Cardiac arrest

44. The effects of the drugs take about 12 hours to wear off properly so that patients' reactions may be slowed during this period; care must be taken in the home as well as on the roads

45. Preferably none without asking the anaesthetist or dental surgeon. For most adults one or two soluble paracetamol at 4-hour intervals would be safe

Sedation

46. What is meant by sedation in dentistry?

47. How may sedation be administered to the patient?

48. Why should the DA learn monitoring and resuscitation techniques before assisting at a sedation or anaesthetic session?

49. How can the DA monitor the patient under sedation?

50. What pre-operative check should the DA make with the patient before sedation?

51. When and what should the patient eat or drink before sedation?

52. Why is it not necessary to have a prolonged period of nil by mouth before sedation?

53. Why should the patient lie flat when sedation is being administered?

54. What is meant by amnesia?

55. Why does the effect of intravenous (i.v.) drugs wear off?

56. Patients should be warned that after i.v. diazepam they may feel sleepy again 6–8 hours after the sedation; why is this?

57. What is a haematoma?

58. How can the DA help to prevent the development of a haematoma?

Sedation

46. The use of drugs to soothe and calm the emotions, enabling treatment to be carried out while retaining verbal contact with the patient. As a result of the sedation the pain threshold may be raised

47. Orally, by inhalation or intravenously and it can be given rectally

48. Trained assistance is important in the smooth running of the session, by helping to prevent emergencies and dealing with them

49. (a) Respiration−feel exhaled air from nose or observe chest movements
(b) Pulse−notice or feel the carotid pulse in the neck or feel the radial pulse in the wrist
(c) Check facial skin for signs of sweating, and colour (pallor or cyanosis)

50. (a) Confirm person's name
(b) Check no cough or cold
(c) When he/she last took food and last took drink
(d) What arrangements the patient has made for getting home, including escort

51. A light meal and a non-alcoholic drink about 2 hours before. This reduces the chances of the patient feeling faint

52. The patients are not anaesthetized; they therefore have control of their reflexes, including those of the larynx

53. (a) It is the natural position for relaxation and the even weight distribution reduces discomfort
(b) This position helps to ensure good oxygenation of the brain
(c) It is easier to give the inhalation or intravenous agent
(d) The patient is ready in the working position

54. Sudden and complete inability to remember events. This is a side-effect of the period of the sedation which the patient welcomes

55. Initially the drugs are concentrated in the brain; they then spread around the body and start to be broken down before excretion

56. Some of the drug is reabsorbed by the brain during excretion

57. When blood leaks from a vessel into the surrounding tissues

58. By making sure that firm pressure is applied over the venepuncture site for 2 minutes after withdrawal of the needle

59. What are the postoperative instructions for the recovery period, when conservation only will be performed using an i.v. sedation technique?

60. What is relative analgesia (RA)?

61. How does RA differ from gaseous general anaesthesia?

62. What are the advantages of RA over i.v. sedation?

63. What hazards to the dental team arise from the use of RA?

64. How may this hazard be reduced?

65. Why might local analgesia be used with RA?

66. Why might i.v. sedation be preferred to RA?

67. What is the immediate recovery period from sedation?

68. What instructions should be given to a patient after sedation?

59. (a) Not to drive cars or to use machinery that day.
    (b) To arrange that the patient is accompanied home by a responsible adult
    (c) That the patient may remain drowsy for some hours
    (d) For this reason they should not be left alone

60. A technique of giving nitrous oxide and oxygen to patients to produce a psychological state which helps to eliminate fear. General anaesthesia cannot be achieved using this technique

61. In RA
    (a) the patient remains conscious and can talk, cough etc.
    (b) a minimum of 30% oxygen is administered
    In GA
    (a) the patient is unconscious
    (b) usually 25–30% oxygen is administered
    (c) other agents e.g. halothane are given

62. (a) More rapid recovery
    (b) Avoids the use of needles
    (c) Avoids the potential hazard of drugs which have to be broken down by the body

63. Nitrous oxide pollution

64. By use of anti-pollution equipment or a well-ventilated room

65. Many patients find inadequate analgesia with RA alone

66. (a) The patient's fear of a mask
    (b) Deeper sedation needed
    (c) Greater control over the dose received by the patient

67. The period during which the patient is not fit to leave the practice. The sedationist should advise on the length of this time

68. Verbally none, as memory will be impaired. Printed instructions should have been given at an earlier appointment; the most important can be given verbally to the person accompanying the patient home

Children's dentistry

Questions

1. What are the primary aims of children's dentistry?
2. What is the most common dental reason for an uncooperative child in the surgery?
3. How can the DA help in introducing a child to the surgery?
4. What are the most important aspects of dentistry for a 2½-year-old child?
5. What advice should be given about teeth to the parents of young children?
6. At what age should brushing of children's teeth start?
7. What is the value of the diet sheet in prevention of dental disease?
8. What advice should be given regarding tooth cleaning for young children?
9. When do the following teeth usually (a) start to calcify, and (b) start to erupt:
    (i) deciduous central incisor?
    (ii) permanent central incisor?
    (iii) permanent first molar?
    (iv) first premolar?

Answers

1. To improve the standard of oral health in the community through:
   (a) a preventive regime and attitude
   (b) willing and co-operative acceptance of dentistry

2. Fear of dentistry based on real or imagined past experience of the patient or of friends or family

3. (a) By helping to create a calm, relaxed and friendly atmosphere
   (b) When bringing patient to the surgery explain what is going to happen using appropriate language; lack of knowledge increases fear

4. (a) To give the parents dental preventive advice
   (b) To allow the child to become familiar with the dentist, the staff and the equipment
   (c) Treatment, if any, is likely to be simple and should encourage patient co-operation

5. (a) Diet control
   (b) Toothbrushing–method and frequency
   (c) Use of fluoride toothpaste
   (d) If necessary, use of fluoride tablets or after the age of 7 years, the use of fluoride mouthwashes
   (e) The importance of keeping the deciduous teeth until natural loss

6. As soon as the first tooth has erupted. This introduces the preventive approach at the earliest opportunity which the child accepts as normal

7. An accurately completed 3 or 4 day sheet shows the full range, content and frequency of intake. Verbal replies tend to correspond to what the patient believes the dentist wishes to hear

8. (a) Small child-size brush, simple technique, flavour of toothpaste which child finds pleasant and preferably containing fluoride
   (b) Cleaning after breakfast and before bed
   (c) Make it a happy procedure; firmness without friction
   (d) Give the child the opportunity to start the cleaning

9. (a) (i) Sixth week intra-uterine
       (ii) At birth
       (iii) At birth
       (iv) 4 years
   (b) (i) 6 months
       (ii) 6 years
       (iii) 6 years
       (iv) 10 years

10. How do enamel and dentine of deciduous teeth differ from these tissues in permanent teeth?

11. How can fluoride be applied to teeth?

12. What are fissure sealants?

13. Why are fissure sealants used?

14. How can the DA help to ensure the successful application of fissure sealants?

15. What are the most common sites for caries before the age of 4 years?

16. How can the dental surgeon detect caries interproximally in deciduous molar teeth?

17. What is rampant caries?

18. For what reasons are carious deciduous molar teeth conserved?

19. What is the usual explanation for extensive caries in deciduous incisors?

20. Why is it less common in lower incisors?

21. Why is the comforter at night particularly bad for teeth?

22. What is the first stage in the treatment of patients with extensive caries?

23. What advice should be given to a child following use of local anaesthesia?

24. Why is pulp size important in the treatment of deciduous teeth?

25. Why is it difficult to root fill completely a deciduous molar tooth?

26. What is meant by pulp mummification?

27. How can a grossly carious deciduous molar tooth best be restored?

10. Each layer is thinner. Enamel is whiter

11. (a) By the patient, in toothpastes and mouthwashes
(b) By the dentist, therapist or hygienist, in a gel or sol used in preformed trays, or in a varnish containing fluoride

12. Plastic materials used to seal naturally occurring pits and fissures in teeth

13. They help to prevent the onset of caries in the most common sites

14. (a) By preparing all equipment, instruments and materials beforehand
(b) Assisting in moisture control
(c) Passing instruments and materials efficiently

15. Occlusal and approximal surfaces of molar teeth

16. Using a probe, by transillumination or by child-size bite-wing radiographs

17. Caries of rapid onset and spread leading to early involvement of the pulp. It affects tooth surfaces usually regarded as immune to caries

18. (a) Prevention of extension of caries
(b) Prevention of pain and infection
(c) Space maintenance for permanent successors

19. Use of a comforter, dummy or feeding bottle with acidic diluted fruit juices, or sucrose-containing drinks, available on demand night and day

20. There is more saliva in this area to wash away the sucrose and to dilute and buffer the acid produced

21. The flow of saliva at night is reduced

22. Correction of dietary faults, usually frequent high intake of sugars

23. Not to bite the numb tissue nor to take hot drinks–give patient the reasons why they should be careful

24. Relative to tooth size it is large and caries soon involves the pulp

25. Because the root canals are fine and curved

26. A method of killing the pulp of a tooth by sealing certain chemicals in the pulp chamber in contact with the remaining vital pulp

27. (a) Endodontic treatment is usually necessary
(b) A stainless steel crown is likely to prove more permanent than amalgam
(c) An alternative is glass ionomer cement

28. If 'tender loving care' does not produce sufficient co-operation to complete necessary treatment, what other options are available?

29. What are the disadvantages of general anaesthesia for children?

30. How can deciduous teeth lead to malocclusion in the permanent dentition?

31. What are the reasons for carrying out orthodontic treatment?

32. What long-term damage to the dentition can occur following accidental trauma, as for example to a deciduous upper incisor?

33. What damage may occur directly to permanent incisor teeth from accidental injury?

34. When a patient contacts the surgery after accidental tooth trauma, what should the DA do?

35. What advice should be given about a permanent tooth which has been knocked out?

36. What is the importance of early treatment of tooth trauma?

37. What tests would the dental surgeon apply to traumatized permanent anterior teeth and why would these tests be used?

38. Why do some teeth discolour after trauma?

39. Why is it difficult to obtain a good apical seal when root filling any of the permanent incisors of a seven year old child?

28. Oral sedation or relative analgesia. General anaesthesia is needed for only a very small percentage of children, except where there is infection

29. (a) There is a medical risk attached to all general anaesthetics
   (b) Many children find it an unpleasant experience, despite the efforts of the anaesthetist
   (c) The experience may put the child off further treatment for years

30. (a) Premature loss of deciduous teeth can lead to loss of space for the permanent successors
   (b) Prolonged retention may cause irregularities

31. (a) To improve appearance and reduce the risk of damage to prominent anterior teeth
   (b) By correcting irregularity to help reduce the incidence of caries and periodontal disease
   (c) To align teeth prior to restorative procedures

32. Damage to the developing successor such as hypoplasia

33. (a) Fracture of some or all of the crown
   (b) Fracture of the root
   (c) Displacement, either total loss or movement within the tooth socket
   (d) Pulp death

34. Arrange an appointment as soon as possible, ideally straight away.

35. (a) Collect the tooth, if dirty then rinse under gentle cold running water
   (b) Place tooth in a buccal sulcus for storage in saliva or in milk in a small container
   (c) Come to the surgery immediately

36. (a) Relief of pain
   (b) Reduction of consequences e.g. cover exposed pulp

37. (a) Visual–to observe tooth displacement, fractures or chipping of tooth crown and any soft-tissue damage
   (b) Palpation–to detect mobility
   (c) Electrical or thermal–to check vitality of the tooth
   (d) Radiographic–to detect tooth displacement or root fracture

38. The pulp bleeds and the residual blood breaks down. The decomposition products stain the dentine, in a manner similar to a bruise. In permanent teeth the pulp frequently dies

39. The root is not fully formed, and the canal will have a wide open apex

40. What is meant by a vital pulpotomy?
41. Why is a pulpotomy carried out?
42. Why replace a tooth lost by trauma?
43. What types of replacement are available to fill such a space?
44. How might loss of one-third of a permanent anterior tooth crown be replaced?
45. Why are permanent jacket crowns not usually placed before the patient has reached 16 years of age?
46. What is a mouth guard?
47. When is a mouth guard worn?
48. Why are they worn?

40. Removal of the pulp tissue from the crown of a tooth

41. To enable the root formation to continue and the apex to close

42. For appearance and to maintain the space

43. An acrylic partial denture or an adhesive bridge. At a later date these might be replaced by a chrome-cobalt denture or a conventional bridge

44. Usually by an acid-etch retained composite

45. (a) On eruption the pulp chamber is large, as time passes there is an increasing thickness of dentine resulting in a smaller pulp chamber and by the age of 16–18 years the risk of exposure or of pulp damage during crown preparation is reduced
   (b) The permanent teeth continue to erupt until about this age which would expose the artificial crown/tooth junction making replacement necessary

46. Usually a soft vinyl plastic horseshoe made to fit over the person's upper teeth

47. When taking part in any 'contact' sports e.g. hockey, rugby, boxing

48. To help to protect the teeth, especially the upper incisors, from trauma

Orthodontics

Questions

1. What is the meaning of the word 'orthodontics'?
2. What does the orthodontist study?
3. What is the purpose of orthodontics?
4. Define 'malocclusion'
5. Give some of the causes of malocclusion
6. What percentage of children have some sort of orthodontic problem?
7. Give some of the reasons for carrying out orthodontics
8. What are the contra-indications to orthodontic treatment?
9. What factors influence the position of teeth in the jaws?
10. Define the following:
    (a) overjet
    (b) overbite
    (c) overcrowding
    (d) cross-bite
11. Briefly, what is meant by a Class I, II and III incisor relationship?

Answers

1. From the Greek words meaning 'straight teeth'

2. (a) The growth and development of teeth, jaws and face
(b) The function of the oral and facial soft tissues
(c) The diagnosis and treatment of malocclusion

3. Prevention or correction of irregularities of tooth position to maintain or preserve the dentition. Adults as well as children are treated

4. A condition in which the teeth are abnormally related

5. (a) Hereditary, e.g. large teeth and small jaws
(b) Premature loss or prolonged retention of deciduous teeth
(c) Digit sucking
(d) Soft tissue behaviour e.g. tongue thrusting

6. Generally considered to be about 50% in UK

7. (a) Aesthetics e.g. irregularity leading to disfigurement, prominence of upper incisors leading to traumatic damage
(b) Functional e.g. teeth damaging opposing soft tissue, food stagnation around irregular teeth, inability to close lips
(c) In association with prosthetic or crown and bridge treatment or with jaw surgery

8. Low patient motivation, poor oral hygiene, high level of dental disease

9. (a) Muscles of the lips, cheeks and tongue
(b) Contacts with adjacent and opposing teeth
(c) Genetics
(d) Habits e.g. digit sucking

10. (a) Horizontal distance between the upper and lower incisors
(b) Vertical overlap of the lower anterior teeth by the upper incisors
(c) Insufficient space for the number of teeth present in the jaws to be well aligned
(d) Variation from the normal overlap of the upper teeth over the lower teeth

11. (a) Class I–normal antero-posterior relationship
(b) Class II division i–where upper incisor teeth meet anterior to the normal occlusion with the lower incisors i.e. increased overjet; Class II division ii–the overjet is about normal but the overbite is increased; frequently the upper lateral incisors are more prominent
(c) Class III–the incisors meet edge to edge or are in reverse overjet

12. Give the three essential items which should be put out for orthodontic diagnosis and treatment planning, before the patient is called to the surgery

13. Why is the cephalograph used in orthodontic assessment?

14. How is it possible that teeth can be moved in bone by means of orthodontic appliances?

15. What should the patient and parents understand before orthodontic treatment is started?

16. Why does the orthodontist usually prefer to extract upper first premolar teeth in Class II cases?

17. What is the name given to the fold of tissue joining the upper lip to the gum in the midline?

18. Why might the orthodontist want this tissue removed, and what is the operation called?

19. What is meant by a 'fixed' orthodontic appliance?

20. How is a fixed appliance held in place?

21. List some of the components of a fixed appliance

22. What are the advantages of a fixed appliance?

23. What are the disadvantages of a fixed appliance?

12. (a) Patient's notes
  (b) Radiographs
  (c) Study models

13. It is a standard and fixed view which is repeatable so that measurements can be made to show changes during and after treatment

14. Bone is a living tissue and is able to be moulded. The bone is resorbed on one side of the tooth socket and new bone is laid down on the other side of the socket

15. Outline of treatment including:
  (a) whether any extractions are needed and which teeth
  (b) nature of appliances, number and frequency of visits
  (c) importance of wearing appliances as prescribed
  (d) need to attend for adjustments
  (e) probable length of course of treatment
  (f) importance of maintaining good oral hygiene and regular dental checks

16. (a) It creates space near the front of the arches to allow the upper anterior teeth to be retracted
  (b) Extractions further back would mean moving more teeth, which would prolong treatment

17. Labial frenum

18. Sometimes it is associated with a space between the upper permanent incisors and it is removed to assist closure of the space; frenectomy

19. An appliance attached directly to the teeth which cannot be removed by the patient

20. (a) Stainless steel bands cemented to the teeth
  (b) Brackets bonded to teeth by an etched composite technique

21. Stainless steel bands, brackets, arch wires, auxiliary springs, elastics

22. (a) Continuous application of forces because patient cannot forget to wear appliance
  (b) More complex tooth movements can be made than with a removable appliance
  (c) Higher quality end-result

23. (a) Special training of operator in techniques
  (b) High cost of materials and chairside time
  (c) A very co-operative patient e.g able to use elastics, able to detect problems such as a loose band
  (d) Appearance of appliance may be more noticeable

24. What instructions are given to patients after fitting a fixed appliance?

25. List the types of removable appliances

26. What are the following:
    (a) a crib?
    (b) a labial bow?
    (c) a spring?

27. What are the advantages of a removable appliance ?

28. What are the disadvantages of a removable appliance?

29. What instructions are given to the patient after fitting a removable appliance?

30. Why do some orthodontic patients wear headgear linked to their appliance?

31. What items should be laid out for fit of a removable appliance appointment?

32. What does the operator check at adjustment appointments?

24. (a) Discomfort may be expected in the first few days
    (b) To return if anything becomes loose or breaks
    (c) Importance of maintaining a very high standard of oral hygiene
    (d) To avoid sticky foods

25. (a) Active simple removable, myofunctional
    (b) Passive retainers, space maintainers

26. (a) A stainless steel wire bent to grip a tooth to help retain a removable appliance
    (b) A stainless steel wire around the labial surface of several anterior teeth, either to help retain the appliance or to move back the anterior teeth
    (c) A flexible stainless steel wire designed to move individual teeth

27. (a) Made in the laboratory and so saves surgery time
    (b) Easy for operator to adjust
    (c) Easy for patient to clean
    (d) Advantages in appearance
    (e) Cheaper to construct

28. (a) Patient is able to mishandle it, bending wires or breaking the appliance
    (b) Patient can leave it out, damage or lose it
    (c) Limitations to tooth movements which can be carried out e.g. whole tooth movements or rotations need a fixed appliance

29. (a) Wear it all the time unless the operator advises otherwise
    (b) Eating and talking may be different for the first day
    (c) Avoid sticky foods
    (d) Clean it carefully after all meals and before going to bed
    (e) Arrange to return to the surgery as soon as possible if teeth hurt or the appliance breaks or rubs
    (f) Do not interfere with the wires on the appliance
    (g) Keep appointments for adjustment

30. This gives reinforced anchorage to prevent forward movement of teeth

31. Patient's notes, new appliance, suitable orthodontic pliers, handpiece and acrylic trimmers, wax pencil, dividers, articulating paper, written instructions for patient; models and radiographs should be available

32. (a) Oral hygiene
    (b) Stability of anchorage teeth
    (c) Amount and direction of tooth movement since last visit
    (d) State of the appliance e.g. cracks, distorted wires
    (e) Retention of cribs
    (f) Activation of springs

33. Give some common reasons why an appliance may not be worn

34. After tooth movements have been completed the patient has to continue to wear an appliance–why is this ?

35. What is the name given to this period of inactive treatment?

36. What is meant in orthodontics by 'relapse'?

37. How can a patient be responsible for poor tooth movement with a removable appliance?

33. (a) Appearance
    (b) Speech or eating problems
    (c) Lost motivation
    (d) Pain or discomfort

34. Until reorganization of bone and the periodontal membrane has taken place. Teeth can easily relapse towards their original position, especially rotated teeth

35. Retention

36. When, after treatment, teeth return towards their original position

37. (a) Not wearing as advised
    (b) Springs worn on wrong side of the tooth
    (c) Distorted or broken spring not noticed

Conservation

Questions

1. The earliest carious lesion can be arrested without the need to restore a tooth–how can this be encouraged by
   (a) the patient?
   (b) the operator?

2. How can patients prolong the life of dental restorations?

3. What are the objectives when restoring a carious lesion?

4. What is meant by the process of micro-leakage of dental restorations?

5. Give five reasons for restoring a tooth

6. Why are temporary fillings used?

7. What are the advantages in using a rubber dam when working on a tooth?

8. What factors does the operator consider when shaping a tooth cavity?

Answers

1. (a) (i) By altering the dietary causative factors e.g. reducing frequency of sugar intake
      (ii) General improved plaque control and use of a fluoride toothpaste with special attention to risk sites
      (iii) Possibly the use of fluoride mouthwashes
   (b) (i) Making sure patient can effectively carry out plaque control
      (ii) Application of topical fluoride to risk sites
      (iii) Advice on diet

2. By maintaining good oral hygiene and having regular dental checks.

3. (a) To remove the carious tooth substance
   (b) To place a restoration which will restore appearance and function as well as prevent recurrence of caries and maintain healthy gingiva

4. There is a microscopic space between the tooth and the restoration, into which fluids and micro-organisms may pass. Corrosion of the restoration occurs which may show as discoloration. Amalgam corrosion products form a seal in the micro-space which helps to reduce further micro-leakage

5. (a) Restoration of function
   (b) Prevention of pain
   (c) Restoration of appearance
   (d) Maintenance of a healthy pulp
   (e) Prevention of further decay

6. (a) To relieve or prevent pain
   (b) To prevent food lodging in the cavity
   (c) To prevent or reduce gingival overgrowth
   (d) To seal in special dressings

7. (a) Barrier against moisture
   (b) Prevents patient from inhaling or ingesting instruments, debris or materials
   (c) Helps to retract the gingiva

8. (a) Elimination of existing decay
   (b) Conservation of hard tissue and pulp
   (c) Elimination of stagnation areas to reduce the recurrence of caries
   (d) Retention of the restoration
   (e) Strength of the restoration

9. Operators try not to remove too much tooth structure during cavity preparation–why is this?

10. Repairing defective restorations is now more common–what are the advantages of this procedure?

11. In tooth preparation, why is enamel usually removed by use of the high-speed drill?

12. Why is water spray used with high-speed burs?

13. Why are slow-speed steel burs not used at very high speed?

14. Why is dentine easier to cut than enamel using slow-speed steel burs?

15. What are the duties of the DA during cavity preparation?

16. When drying a tooth cavity, why should the DA take care not to over-dry the dentine?

17. Give reasons for the use of cavity linings.

18. How may a tooth cavity be kept free from saliva?

19. Why are calcium hydroxide materials used in deep cavities?

20. What is meant by the term 'pulp capping'?

21. Why does the operator remove all cavity lining from enamel walls before placing the filling material?

22. What is a dentine pin?

23. What is an adhesive restoration?

9. (a) To maintain the natural strength of the tooth
   (b) Small restorations are likely to be stronger than larger ones

10. (a) The sound part of the restoration is untouched and remains so
   (b) Enlargement of the cavity is kept to the minimum
   (c) Retention problems are reduced
   (d) Shortened procedure

11. Enamel is a very hard substance and is not easy to cut with burs in a slow-speed handpiece

12. (a) Protection of the pulp from the heat of cutting
   (b) Removal of cutting debris

13. They would blunt too quickly

14. Dentine is less highly calcified and therefore softer

15. (a) Retraction and protection of the cheek or tongue with suction tip
   (b) Aspiration of saliva, water and debris
   (c) Cavity toilet using 3-in-1 syringe
   (d) Passing of instruments and adjustment of light as required
   (e) Monitoring the patient

16. Desiccation of dentine can lead to after-pain

17. (a) Protection against thermal and chemical irritation
   (b) Therapeutic effect to promote healing of a damaged pulp
   (c) Strengthening of tooth structure by bonding if using glass ionomer cement

18. (a) By use of cotton wool rolls or dry pads plus a saliva ejector or aspirator tip
   (b) Alternatively by use of a rubber dam
   (c) Moisture in the cavity is removed by air from the 3-in-1 syringe

19. (a) They encourage the formation of reparative dentine
   (b) They are alkaline and retard the caries process

20. Covering a small exposed bleeding area of pulp, usually with some form of calcium hydroxide to promote formation of reparative dentine

21. The lining would wear or dissolve away leaving a defect which may lead to further carious attack

22. A piece of special wire which is screwed into dentine to aid retention of fillings. These pins may also be retained by friction or by cement

23. One which bonds directly to the tooth surface

24. Give the advantages of adhesive restorations

25. How are very large amalgam fillings retained?

26. Why are matrix bands and strips fitted to teeth?

27. Why are wood or plastic wedges used during placement of fillings?

28. How can the DA help to ensure that a metal matrix will fit a tooth accurately?

29. What are the duties of the DA in relation to amalgam matrix holders and bands?

30. Give the reasons why an operator may use dental floss between two teeth in a patient's mouth

31. Give four factors which influence the operator's choice of filling materials

32. What is meant by a 'plastic' filling material?

33. What are the advantages of silver amalgam as a filling material?

34. What is the main disadvantage to the patient of amalgam as a filling material?

35. Name the types of amalgam alloy available (not trade names)

24. (a) Minimum tooth preparation needed
  (b) A physical seal is formed between the tooth and the restoration

25. By use of undercut dentine supplemented by dentine pins. A gold veneer crown fitted over the tooth and amalgam adds to retention

26. (a) To assist during condensation of the filling material
  (b) To help shape the filling to the tooth and cavity shape
  (c) To ensure that the filling gets maximum retention from the cavity shape
  (d) To help produce a smooth surface
  (e) To reduce the amount of excess filling at the edges of the restoration

27. To improve the fit of the matrix band or strip against the interproximal surface of the tooth at the gingival margin

28. (a) Remove all debris before sterilization
  (b) Check for damage and replace the matrix strip if it is damaged

29. (a) Before handing to the operator, adjust band for correct quadrant and approximate tooth size
  (b) After use, clean thoroughly, check for damage and replace band as necessary. Full sterilization is needed as the band may have been in contact with blood

30. (a) To demonstrate flossing technique
  (b) To check for rough edges of restorations or calculus
  (c) To clean between teeth to aid diagnosis
  (d) To help take rubber dam through the contact point

31. (a) Size of the cavity
  (b) Amount of tooth crown remaining
  (c) Position of the cavity in the tooth and in the mouth
  (d) The quality of the patient's oral hygiene

32. A material which is soft or plastic when placed and which hardens on setting

33. (a) Strong enough to withstand masticatory forces of most patients
  (b) Easily handled
  (c) Relatively cheap

34. Appearance

35. (a) Conventional: lathe cut, these have irregular shaped particles; spherical, less mercury needed and the round particles pack together more densely
  (b) High copper: about 12%

36. Some modern amalgam alloys contain a higher proportion of copper–what advantages does this give?

37. Why is hand mixing of silver amalgam seldom used nowadays?

38. Refilling or re-use of prepacked amalgam capsules is not advised–why is this?

39. What are the effects on the DA of the handling of amalgam?

40. Why should waste amalgam be stored under water?

41. Why does the operator 'condense' the amalgam into the cavity?

42. When packing a plastic filling material the operator is careful not to leave any gaps between the material and the cavity margin–why is this?

43. Why should amalgam be used immediately after mixing?

44. What are the results of excess mercury in an amalgam restoration?

45. What will be the result of moisture contamination of amalgam?

46. Why are the occlusal surfaces of fillings carved to the tooth contour?

47. What are the reasons for carving an amalgam filling?

48. How can the DA help the operator during amalgam carving?

36. (a) Less corrosion
    (b) Reduced chance of margin fracture

37. (a) Mercury hazard is reduced by the mechanical method
    (b) Mechanical method is faster
    (c) Mechanical method produces a more consistent mix

38. Unless the capsule join can be effectively sealed a fine spray of mercury droplets may escape during mixing

39. Mercury may be absorbed through the skin, leading to mercury poisoning

40. To reduce the risk of mercury vaporization

41. (a) To adapt it to the internal cavity shape for retention
    (b) To reduce deficiencies at the cavity margins
    (c) To reduce the amount of mercury in the filling and so increase the strength of the restoration
    (d) To reduce air spaces which lead to weakness and at the surface plaque accumulation

42. (a) Voids can lead to sensitivity and recurrent caries
    (b) These gaps can result in weakness of the filling

43. It will start to set and if there is undue delay the amalgam will be weaker (a 5-minute delay could make it 40% weaker)

44. The set amalgam is weaker. It is more likely that the restoration will break or that the edges will break away

45. There will be excessive expansion resulting in :
    (a) a protruding restoration; secondary caries may start at the overhanging margins
    (b) pressure within the tooth leading to pain
    (c) expansion can lead to fracture of part of the tooth e.g. a cusp

46. (a) To prevent damage to that tooth, the filling and to the opposing tooth by premature contact
    (b) To allow full masticatory function

47. (a) To achieve the correct level for occlusion. This prevents damage to the filling from premature contact with the opposing teeth
    (b) To shape it for correct masticatory function

48. (a) Passing instruments
    (b) Aspiration of debris
    (c) Insertion of articulating paper, in a holder, between the occlusal surfaces as requested by the operator

49. After an amalgam restoration has been placed, what advice should be given to the patient about (a) short-term and (b) longer-term care of the filling?

50. A few days after placement of a restoration the patient may complain of food packing between that tooth and the adjacent one—why might this happen?

51. What are the reasons for polishing fillings?

52. List instruments and materials for polishing an amalgam filling

53. In simple terms, what are the constituents of composite filling materials?

54. What are the advantages of composites over other anterior restorative materials?

55. What causes composite filling materials to set?

56. How can the setting time of 'two paste' composites be retarded?

57. Composites should not be mixed with stainless steel spatulas—why not?

58. On the other hand, stainless steel instruments are used to place the composite material into the cavity—why is this?

59. Despite the very hard particles composite fillings do very slowly wear away—why does this occur?

60. What is the effect of room light on light-cured composites?

61. How can this effect be kept to a minimum?

49. (a) (i) Not to bite on it for at least 4 hours, longer for some alloys
   (ii) To return if any discomfort persists after 48 hours
   (b) (i) Maintain good oral hygiene and diet control to prevent deterioration of the restoration
   (ii) Regular checks to detect and treat any recurrent caries or damage to the restoration

50. (a) A piece of filling may have broken away
   (b) There is a poor contact with the adjacent tooth

51. (a) Improved aesthetics
   (b) Better marginal adaptation
   (c) Reduced plaque adherence following:
      (i) removal of any rough and overhanging edges
      (ii) elimination of surface defects
         production of a smooth surface

52. Smoothed with smoothing stones, finishing burs, discs and strips
   Polished with special polishing points or paste on brush or rubber cup
   Materials—pumice powder, glycerin or fluoride gel, zinc oxide, methylated spirits
   Both the high-speed and slow-speed handpieces should be available

53. Glass particles and a plastic bonding resin

54. (a) They are almost insoluble in oral fluids
   (b) They are very hard and resistant to wear
   (c) There is good colour matching
   (d) Their properties of expansion and contraction are similar to those of teeth
   (e) They can be used with the acid-etch technique

55. A catalyst, either chemical or light

56. By use of a lower proportion of catalyst

57. The hard glass particles rub off some of the metal during the relatively long mixing time, resulting in a grey colour

58. The composite material is only being pushed or wiped into the cavity with minimum friction between instrument, composite and tooth. Teflon instruments are available for composite placement.

59. The resin is relatively soft and wears, with the result that the glass particles fall away

60. They start to set

61. (a) Replace the lid after taking amount needed
   (b) Until needed, composite should be covered to exclude light
   (c) Turn away operating light

62. Why should the shade used for filling materials be noted?

63. Why does the colour of a tooth-coloured filling sometimes appear to vary during the day?

64. Composite fillings closely match a variety of tooth shades–why is this?

65. Some chemical cure composite restorations may become discoloured–why does this occur?

66. Why should composite filling materials be stored in a cool place?

67. Why should the excess material be left on the pad?

68. Why are diamond burs preferred for removing composites?

69. Why have special posterior composites been developed?

70. Why do composite fillings need a lining?

71. What is the effect of etching dentine?

72. Why should eugenol-containing linings not be mixed for placement directly under composite fillings?

73. Why is the acid-etch technique used with composite restorations?

74. What is the etchant and what precautions should be taken?

75. What tissue is acid etching meant to affect?

76. What is the appearance of etched enamel?

77. What effect does etching have on that tissue?

78. Why is this effect needed?

79. In simple terms, what do glass ionomer materials contain?

80. Glass ionomer restorations stay in place on flat surfaces–how are they retained?

81. Why is a conditioner used before placement of glass ionomer fillings?

62. Easy reference in future; if not good, then not used next time

63. The shade is modified under different lighting conditions

64. The glass particles with a natural tooth background colour reflect light which is tooth coloured

65. The surface roughens and the resin stains, causing the restorations to go yellow

66. An increase in temperature shortens the shelf-life of the material

67. To check setting of the material

68. The filler is very hard and blunts all burs, but diamond least of all

69. To resist the heavy abrasion which occurs during mastication

70. To prevent pulpal irritation from
(a) the etching medium, liquid or gel
(b) chemicals in the composite material

71. Irritation of the dentinal tubules resulting in after-pain. It is important to provide conditioner, not etchant, for the operator

72. The eugenol affects the composite making it softer

73. (a) As an aid to retention
(b) To eliminate marginal leakage

74. (a) 35–50% phosphoric acid
(b) As it is a strong acid care must be taken not to get it on the skin or mucosa. Any misplaced drops should be removed and the area copiously irrigated with water. There is less risk if the gel form is used

75. Enamel

76. A white opaque area

77. It creates a microscopically porous surface

78. Composite material can flow into this surface which, on setting, forms a strong mechanical bond of thousands of little tags of composite in enamel

79. Glass particles and polyacrylic acid. For use in posterior teeth fine amalgam particles are also included, the material is called a 'cermet'

80. A chemical bond occurs between the material and calcium of the tooth

81. (a) It removes any plaque or grease from the surface, but it does not etch
(b) It improves the bonding to dentine

82. Why is a lining not normally placed under glass ionomer material?

83. Why is glass ionomer cement sometimes used to line composite fillings?

84. Accurate dispensing of drop size is important for the correct mixing of some materials. How best can this be achieved?

85. What should glass ionomer fillings be covered with immediately after insertion? Give the reasons for this covering

86. Give the advantages of glass ionomer as a filling material

82. (a) Glass ionomer is not irritant to the pulp unless the dentine is very thin or newly cut
(b) Retention of the material comes from the bonding to dentine

83. For added retention of the composite which can bond to glass ionomer

84. (a) Hold the container away from the mixing surface to allow free dropping
(b) Rubber dropper type–squeeze the bulb slowly
(c) Tube type–invert the container and let the warmth of the hand expand the air in the container; this forces out full-size drops

85. Petroleum jelly or copal varnish, to keep out moisture. Moisture contamination reduces adhesion to the tooth; in addition, the material may crumble

86. (a) Retention by chemical bonding to tooth structure, reducing the need to shape the cavity for mechanical retention
(b) Reduced micro-leakage due to bonding to tooth
(c) Fluoride can pass from the material into enamel, helping to inhibit caries

Endodontics

Questions

1. What is meant by the word 'endodontics'?
2. What are the basic objectives of root canal treatment?
3. Why might carious dentine be deliberately left in a tooth?
4. What is meant by pulp capping?
5. How can the vitality of a tooth be tested?
6. In an unfilled tooth, what does a discoloured natural crown usually indicate?
7. What are the main causes of pulpitis?
8. What is the commonest cause of a periapical abscess?
9. Why is a tooth with a periapical abscess tender to pressure?
10. How can the pulp of an infected tooth sometimes still be vital?
11. What is the method of sterilizing root canal instruments?
12. How can the following be sterilized in the surgery:
    (a) paper points?
    (b) gutta percha (g.p.) points?
13. Give four reasons for the use of a rubber dam in endodontics
14. How may a root canal be kept dry and free from contamination if a rubber dam is not used?
15. When should a safety chain be attached to root canal instruments?
16. Why are radiographs taken before starting endodontic treatment?

Answers

1. 'Endo' meaning 'in', therefore inside tooth treatment. This will include all forms of pulp therapy–mummification, pulpotomy, pulpectomy, etc.

2. To render the tooth free from pain and infection. This will, in turn, prevent further infection of the periapical area from the root canal

3. To avoid a carious exposure and damage to the pulp

4. Techniques whereby an attempt is made to preserve the vitality of a tooth with pulp damage. Usually calcium hydroxide is applied to the dentine and pulp before placement of a restoration

5. By use of an electric pulp tester, warmed gutta percha, ethyl chloride spray on cotton wool, drilling into dentine without analgesia

6. That the tooth is dead following trauma

7. (a) Irritation due to chemical and thermal changes
   (b) Infection, usually caries
   (c) Trauma

8. A non-vital pulp, usually attributable to caries

9. The inflammatory exudate causes pressure on the nerve endings in the periodontal ligament

10. The pulp contains numerous nerve fibres most of which will be dead in an infected pulp, but some nerve fibres could still be alive

11. The full autoclave or dry-heat sterilizing cycle

12. (a) Dry heat at 140°C for three hours (this prevents charring) or 160°C for 1 hour. Autoclaving is suitable only if the cycle includes a drying phase
    (b) Chemical disinfectants

13. (a) To reduce the risk of contamination of the root canal by oral bacteria
    (b) To keep the teeth dry
    (c) To control irrigation liquid
    (d) To prevent inhalation or swallowing of instruments

14. By the use of cotton wool rolls, absorbent pads and efficient suction

15. When a rubber dam is not being used

16. (a) As an aid to diagnosis
    (b) To indicate the shape of the root canals and any obstruction
    (c) To help indicate the chances of successful root treatment
    (d) As a guide to root length

17. What are the four important stages in root canal therapy?

18. What is meant by an access cavity?

19. What instruments should be laid out to prepare an access cavity?

20. What is the use of a glass-bead sterilizer?

21. Indicate the limitations of the glass-bead sterilizer

22. In endodontics what are the uses of the following:
    (a) smooth broaches
    (b) barbed broaches?

23. List the types of
    (a) root canal reamers
    (b) root canal files

24. What is a 'combination' root instrument?

25. What is the action of the giromatic handpiece?

26. Give two advantages of giromatic instruments.

27. Give two disadvantages of giromatic instruments

28. What are the uses of the following:
    (a) reamers?
    (b) root canal files?

29. Why should a root canal be shaped carefully?

17. (a) Elimination of caries, opening pulp chamber and removal of pulp debris
    (b) Preparation of the root canal
    (c) Elimination of sepsis
    (d) Filling of the root canal

18. It is the aperture made in the crown of the tooth to reach the root canals

19. (a) Rubber dam equipment
    (b) Air turbine and suitable burs
    (c) Low-speed drill and burs
    (d) Mirror and probe
    (e) Suction equipment

20. To disinfect root canal instruments during treatment of a patient e.g. between canals

21. It is not a means of sterilization between patients as time and temperature are inadequate–250°C for 10 seconds

22. (a) Finding and exploring root canals. They can be used with radiographs to determine the length of a root canal
    (b) Removal of pulp tissue, paper points or cotton wool from the root canal

23. (a) (i) engine–rotary and giromatic
        (ii) hand reamers
    (b) (i) engine–giromatic
        (ii) hand–K-file, Hedstroem, Unifile

24. An instrument which has the action of both file and reamer e.g. K-flex

25. It oscillates through a right-angle only

26. (a) The fine ones are flexible so that they will adapt to curved canals
    (b) They are less likely than other types of instrument to fracture

27. (a) The range of sizes is limited
    (b) They do not produce a tapered canal to fit g.p. or silver points
    (c) In narrow curved canals they may not follow the curve of the canal and may perforate the wall of the root into the periodontal ligament

28. (a) To clean, shape and straighten the root canal
    (b) (i) to smooth the walls of the root canal
        (ii) to prepare wide curved or irregular-shaped canals

29. To ensure a good fit of the filling point

30. Why is it necessary to clean the walls of root canals?

31. How can the DA help with the preparation of root instruments during treatment?

32. How many root canals are usually found in :
    (a) upper lateral incisor
    (b) upper first premolar
    (c) upper first molar
    (d) lower lateral incisor
    (e) lower first premolar
    (f) lower first permanent molar

33. List the uses of paper points in endodontics

34. What is the danger in using air from the 3 in 1 syringe to dry root canals?

35. Why is the root canal irrigated during instrumentation?

36. What solutions are commonly used to irrigate root canals?

37. Why is it important not to use unsterile instruments in root canals?

38. How can cross-infection during endodontic treatment be prevented?

39. Why are intermediate root dressings inserted?

40. Can the root of a tooth have more than one apical opening?

41. Is the apical foramen always at the apex of a root?

42. How can the operator judge that the g.p. or silver point will reach the root apex?

43. Why is a root sealer used as part of the root filling?

44. Why are g.p. or silver points used when root filling a tooth?

30. Micro-organisms are present in the canal end of dentinal tubules and could re-infect the canal if left in sufficient numbers

31. (a) Setting the measuring stops to the working length
(b) Offering the instruments in size order
(c) Wiping clean, sterilizing in glass-bead sterilizer ready for re-use on the patient

32. (a) 1
(b) 2
(c) at least 3
(d) at least 1
(e) 1
(f) at least 3

33. (a) To absorb blood or pus from the canal
(b) To help to dry the canal
(c) To carry medicaments into the canal

34. Forcing debris or air through the apex. This can usually be avoided by not placing the nozzle in the access cavity

35. (a) To assist in removal of debris
(b) To lubricate and so ease instrumentation
(c) To assist in disinfection

36. Sodium hypochlorite 1000 p.p.m., normal saline

37. Introduction of other micro-organisms would further complicate treatment, especially if they reach the periapical tissues

38. (a) Sterile instrument kit
(b) Use of a rubber dam
(c) Care not to touch the working end of instruments
(d) Resting instruments on a sterile surface or on a stand
(e) Cleaning and sterilization of instruments after use

39. To kill micro-organisms in the root canal

40. Yes

41. No

42. (a) By measurements obtained from a diagnostic radiograph taken with a measuring instrument in the root canal
(b) Using electronic measurement

43. Most root canals are irregular and so the paste is used to fill the space between the canal wall and the points

44. (a) To form, with sealer paste, a complete seal of the main apical foramen
(b) To help push sealer paste into lateral root canals

45. What is a master point?

46. What is a lateral spreader instrument used for?

47. How can paste sealer be carried to the apex of the tooth?

48. Sometimes only the apical third of the root canal is filled–why is this?

49. In which cases might the operator prefer to use a silver point?

50. Why is a radiograph taken of the completed root filling?

51. Why might a course of antibiotics be prescribed when root filling a tooth?

52. Before sterilizing, what should the DA do with root canal instruments?

53. Give two ways in which a periapical abscess may be drained

54. What instructions are given to a patient about mouth care after drainage of an abscess?

55. For what reasons would a dental surgeon extirpate a vital pulp?

56. What is an apicectomy?

57. For what reasons might an apicectomy be carried out?

58. What is meant by a retrograde amalgam?

59. What is meant by endosonics?

45. A g.p. point which fits the apical end of the canal

46. To compress the master g.p. point against part of the canal wall to allow an additional or accessory point to be inserted. This may be repeated several times to obtain a well-compacted root filling

47. By means of a hand reamer rotated in reverse or using a rotary paste filler

48. It is easier to prepare the root canal for a post crown

49. (a) In teeth with very fine canals
(b) In curved root canals

50. (a) To check that a satisfactory root filling has been placed
(b) For comparison against review radiographs taken to show the periapical condition at recall appointments

51. (a) Because of the patient's medical state
(b) To aid the control of periapical infection

52. (a) Make them physically clean
(b) Check their length in case of fracture
(c) Check for any distortion which might lead to fracture during next use
(d) Fine instruments used in curved molar canals may need to be discarded after each case

53. (a) Drainage through the root canal
(b) Incision of the gum

54. (a) Frequent hot salt mouthwashes
(b) Full oral hygiene

55. (a) Following severe trauma
(b) In a small number of cases in crown and bridge work—usually when a tooth is in a slightly abnormal position and pulpal exposure would occur during crown preparation

56. The surgical removal of the apex of a tooth

57. (a) Persistent unresolved infection
(b) Infection at apex of a post-crowned tooth
(c) Overfilling of root canal
(d) Where there is an obstruction in the root canal

58. An amalgam restoration placed at the root apex during an apicectomy. Used to ensure a good apical seal

59. The use of ultrasonic equipment to shape and clean root canals

Crowns, inlays and bridges

Questions

1. List the general advantages of gold as a restorative material
2. Why might a gold inlay be fitted instead of using amalgam to restore a tooth?
3. What is an overlay?
4. What are the advantages of an overlay over an inlay?
5. Briefly, what is the main difference between the indirect and the direct inlay impression techniques in the laboratory?
6. Which materials are commonly used to obtain an indirect impression of an inlay cavity?
7. Why is gingival retraction cord used before an indirect impression is taken?
8. When fitting a gold inlay what does the operator check?
9. Why are the margins of a gold restoration 'burnished'?
10. Define what is meant by a crown restoration
11. List the types of permanent crown
12. List the materials used for permanent crowns
13. What is a metal-ceramic crown?
14. When are metal-ceramic anterior crowns made in preference to porcelain?
15. When are metal-ceramic posterior crowns made instead of gold alone?

Answers

1. (a) Strength
   (b) Does not corrode in the mouth
   (c) Retains a high polish
   (d) Wears away at similar rate to teeth

2. (a) To reduce the risk of fracture of a large restoration
   (b) To fit a difficult cavity shape
   (c) To get a good contact with the adjacent tooth

3. A gold inlay which also covers one or more cusps

4. (a) Reduces the risk of fracture of remaining tooth substance by protecting it from occlusal stress
   (b) As a bridge abutment it is better retained

5. (a) Indirect technique–a model is made from the impression of the tooth and inlay cavity; the gold restoration is made to fit the model
   (b) Direct technique–the impression of the cavity is taken in special wax and cast in metal without any intermediate stages

6. The elastomeric materials e.g. silicones, polyethers

7. (a) To retract the gingiva from the margin of the preparation. This helps to produce an impression with clearly defined gingival margins and helps to lead to a good marginal fit of the restoration
   (b) If necessary, to restrict bleeding from the gingiva at the margin

8. Fit of edges, contacts with adjacent teeth, occlusion with opposing teeth

9. To ensure perfect adaptation to the tooth so reducing micro-leakage

10. A full or partial replacement of the clinical crown of a tooth

11. Full veneer and partial veneer (3/4), either may be on a post and core

12. (a) Anterior–porcelain, metal-ceramic, acrylic
    (b) Posterior–gold, metal-ceramic

13. A crown made of cast metal to which porcelain is fused

14. (a) History of previous fracture of a porcelain crown
    (b) Heavy or a close 'bite'
    (c) As a bridge abutment

15. Usually for sake of appearance e.g. upper premolars

16. Why is it necessary to remove about 1 mm of tooth substance when preparing a tooth for a porcelain crown?

17. Which materials are used to take the detailed impression of a crown or bridge preparation?

18. What are the criteria for a 'good mix' of elastomeric material?

19. After removal of an elastomeric impression from the mouth how should it be cared for?

20. Apart from the instructions and the crown impression, what else does the technician require before making a crown?

21. List the basic instructions which need to be given to the laboratory

22. What factors make it difficult to select porcelain shades accurately?

23. Before crowning, how may extensive loss of tooth substance be replaced?

24. What procedure is carried out before a metal post is made?

25. What is the name of the process used to obtain a gold casting?

26. What basic types of post and core are available for post crowns?

27. Briefly, how are porcelain jacket crowns made in the laboratory?

16. To give adequate thickness of the artificial crown for strength, aesthetics and to allow the natural contour of the tooth to be reproduced

17. One of the elastomeric type or a reversible hydrocolloid

18. (a) No streaks or unmixed material
(b) Free of air bubbles
(c) Mixed within recommended time—usually 45–60 seconds

19. (a) Any blood or saliva should be washed off
(b) The impression should be disinfected and re-washed
(c) It should be dried immediately
(d) Then carefully stored, dry in a plastic bag bearing the patient's name
(e) Sent to the laboratory with instructions

20. (a) An impression of the teeth of the opposing arch
(b) A wax 'bite' wafer to show the relationship of the dental arches

21. (a) Patient's full name
(b) Full details of laboratory work required–tooth, type of restoration, material to be used, shade
(c) Date of next appointment
(d) Name of operator

22. Uncompensated artificial light, direct sunlight, strong surrounding colours, subject not at eye level

23. (a) By use of dentine pins or screws and permanent filling material
After removal of the pulp and achieving a satisfactory apical seal:
(b) By use of one or more precast metal posts
(c) Construction of a cast metal post and core

24. A good root filling must be placed

25. The lost wax process

26. (a) Cast–made to fit each canal
(b) Pre-cast–selected from a range of types and sizes
(c) Direct–fitted wire, cemented into the root canal, on which a core is built in the mouth

27. (a) A model of the crown preparation is covered with thin platinum foil
(b) Damp porcelain powder is painted on to the foil and then fused in a furnace
(c) Further layers of powder are added and fused until the individual shape and shade of the crown is built up
(d) Finally the crown is glazed to produce the smooth outer surface

28. What is meant by a dental lute?

29. List the materials commonly used as lutes

30. Decreasing the powder content of zinc phosphate cement has what effect on the cement?

31. What should be the consistency of the lute for cementation of a crown?

32. What are the probable results of a 'too thick' mix of lute?

33. What are the probable results of a 'high spot' on a crown?

34. List the reasons why temporary crowns are fitted between the preparation and fit appointments

35. List the types of temporary crown

36. Give the reasons for replacing missing natural teeth

37. How can missing natural teeth be replaced?

38. What patient factors are considered before the patient is offered a replacement for missing teeth?

39. What is a dental bridge?

40. Name the parts of a bridge

41. Bridges are usually constructed of which materials?

42. Why do patients particularly like bridges?

43. Define the terms 'abutment' and 'pontic'.

28. A material to fill the micro space between the preparation and the restoration. This used to be called a 'cement' but other types of material are now available

29. Zinc polycarboxylate, zinc phosphate, glass ionomer

30. (a) Makes it flow more easily
(b) Reduces the strength and increases the solubility of the cement

31. Slightly runny but not fluid enough to drop off the spatula

32. The material will not flow easily so that:
(a) The crown will not seat down fully, leading to a raised bite and a poor marginal seal
(b) Excess pressure may need to be used to seat the crown and in the case of a porcelain crown, this may result in fracture of the porcelain

33. (a) A tender tooth
(b) A broken crown
(c) Excess wear of the crown
(d) A 'bite of convenience'
(e) Pain in the temporo-mandibular joint

34. (a) To protect the tooth from irritation e.g. thermal changes
(b) To maintain gingival health
(c) Appearance
(d) Prevention of movement e.g. over-eruption or drifting

35. (a) Anterior–clear celluloid crown form, polycarbonate crown form, a copy of the tooth using resin in an alginate impression
(b) Posterior–metal crown form (aluminium or stainless steel), a copy of the tooth using resin in an alginate impression

36. Appearance, maintenance of remaining dentition, masticatory efficiency, stability of adjacent teeth, speech

37. By partial dentures or bridges

38. Plaque control, control of dental disease, suitable supporting teeth, ability to accept dental treatment, ability to pay

39. An artificial replacement for one or more missing teeth which is supported by other teeth and is usually not removable by the patient

40. Abutments and pontics

41. Gold, porcelain; acrylic facings can be used

42. Confidence that their false tooth does not move causing embarrassment or risk of swallowing

43. An abutment is the tooth which retains the bridge. A pontic is the connector bearing the missing natural tooth

44. What factors are considered before a bridge is designed?

45. What are the advantages of bridges over partial dentures?

46. What is a 'fixed-fixed' bridge?

47. What is an 'adhesive' bridge?

48. What are the advantages of the adhesive bridge over conventional bridges?

49. What materials are used to fix a conventional bridge to supporting teeth?

50. What should be the consistency of these lutes and why?

51. How can the DA increase the working time of the dental lute?

52. What are the reasons for the use of a rubber dam when attaching an adhesive bridge?

53. Why must patients maintain a high standard of plaque control before and after partial dentures or bridges are fitted?

54. Which surface of a bridge is more likely to lead to cleaning problems for the patient?

55. How can the patient best clean this surface?

56. Why might it be difficult to use a toothbrush in this area?

57. Give the reasons for fitting a temporary bridge between visits.

44. Existing restorations, vitality, periapical and periodontal condition of abutment teeth; size of the bridge; general state of the mouth and control of disease; the occlusion

45. (a) They are held firmly in place
   (b) They are usually about the same size as the natural teeth, so cause less interference with speech etc.
   (c) They prevent movement of adjacent teeth

46. A one piece bridge where the retainers are rigidly joined

47. A bridge retained on the abutment teeth by etched composite material

48. (a) Little or no tooth preparation is required
   (b) Simple surgery procedure

49. Luting cements e.g. zinc phosphate, glass ionomer, polycarboxylate

50. Runny so that they only just drip from the mixing spatula. This consistency allows time to seat properly more than one restoration

51. (a) By chilling both the materials and the mixing slab
   (b) By slaking the material. A few grains of powder are added to the liquid which starts the chemical reaction. When the operator is ready more powder is added to make a thin mix which sets more rapidly, but because of low powder content is not as strong as a standard mix

52. (a) Prevention of inhalation of bridge or other items
   (b) Isolation of abutment teeth to control moisture during etching, irrigation and attachment

53. (a) To produce and maintain the best possible periodontal state
   (b) To prevent caries
   (c) For the patient to get the maximum long-term benefit from the prosthesis

54. The mucosal surface of the pontic

55. Using dental floss, possibly superfloss

56. Even an interspace type of brush may be too big to clean between mucosa and pontic unless a 'wash through' design has been used

57. (a) To protect abutment teeth from irritation and damage
   (b) To maintain position of abutment teeth
   (c) To maintain gingival margins
   (d) Appearance

Extractions and minor oral surgery

Questions

1. What are the main reasons for extracting teeth?
2. How many roots do the following teeth commonly possess:
   (a) lower deciduous molars
   (b) upper deciduous molars
   (c) incisors
   (d) lower premolars
   (e) upper first premolars
   (f) upper first permanent molars
   (g) lower second permanent molars

3. Give simple patient instructions to reduce haemorrhage after tooth extraction

4. How does a tooth socket normally heal?

5. What is a 'dry socket'?

6. How can a patient help to cause a dry socket?

7. How does a dry socket heal?

8. Give the principles for the treatment of a dry socket

9. What is the use of a periosteal elevator?

10. Why are patients advised not to rinse, and to avoid raising their blood pressure for 24 hours after an extraction?

Answers

1. Caries, periodontal disease and orthodontic reasons

2. (a) 2
   (b) 3
   (c) 1
   (d) 1
   (e) 2
   (f) 3
   (g) 2

3. (a) No rinsing for 24 hours
   (b) No exercise
   (c) No hot fluids
   (d) No alcohol
   (e) No smoking

4. A blood clot forms to fill the socket. This clot becomes organized initially as granulation tissue, then forming fibrous tissue and new capillaries. Later bone is formed. Epithelium grows across the surface

5. Where there is little or no blood clot in a tooth socket–the bony socket walls become exposed and frequently become infected. There is a great deal of pain and a foul taste

6. By interfering with the formation of the blood clot e.g. rinsing or poking it with the tongue, finger or a foreign body

7. There is virtually no blood clot so that healing takes place from the bone surfaces

8. (a) Irrigate to remove soft debris e.g. sterile water or saline
   (b) Place a sedative dressing e.g. zinc oxide–eugenol bound together with cotton wool or ribbon gauze
   (c) Hot salt mouthwashes to maintain cleanliness and encourage a good blood supply
   (d) Possibly prescribe analgesics and/or antibiotics
   (e) Review to remove dressing after a week, possibly a repeat dressing

9. To lift soft tissue away from the underlying bone. It is sometimes used to retract tissue and to protect tissues when using cutting instruments

10. Rinsing might dislodge the forming blood clot and raised blood pressure might lead to continuous slow bleeding

11. Why are hot salt mouthwashes advised, starting 24 hours after an extraction?

12. What instruments should be laid out for suturing?

13. What materials are used in dental suturing?

14. Why are non-resorbable sutures usually removed after 5–7 days?

15. What instrument might the surgeon use to hold soft tissue when suturing?

16. What are cheatle forceps used for?

17. How should cheatle forceps be stored?

18. How can the DA help to allay the patient's fears?

19. What is meant by minor oral surgery?

20. List some examples of minor oral surgical procedures

21. What is an abscess sinus?

22. What is the commonest cause of a dental abscess in young people?

23. What is an apicectomy?

24. What is a biopsy?

25. What should the DA do with tissue for biopsy?

11. (a) To help keep the socket clean and free from food
    (b) To encourage vasodilatation and hence the healing process

12. Suture pack containing needle holder, tissue forceps, scissors, cheek retractor and sucker

13. (a) Non-resorbable thread made from black silk or types of nylon
    (b) Resorbable thread made from catgut or man-made materials

14. (a) The edges of the wound will have started to heal
    (b) There is little risk of bleeding
    (c) The sutures become loose and irritate the patient
    (d) They are foreign bodies and will lead to an acute inflammatory reaction in the tissues

15. Toothed tissue forceps

16. (a) Removing sterile instruments from the sterilizer
    (b) Removing sterile instruments from their packs when laying up trays and trolleys

17. In a sterile manner–first they should be sterilized then stored in a covered sterile tray. They should only be placed in a freshly made antiseptic solution

18. (a) By explaining in simple terms what is going to happen
    (b) By remaining calm herself, and by reassuring the patient
    (c) By not displaying instruments

19. A procedure in which there is planned cutting of the mucosa

20. (a) Removal of buried teeth, roots or impacted teeth
    (b) Periodontal surgery
    (c) Biopsy
    (d) Apicectomy
    (e) Removal of cysts
    (f) Repair of an oro-antral connection or of a fistula

21. The track along which an abscess has discharged to the surface

22. Caries

23. Surgical removal of the apex of a tooth

24. The surgical removal of a piece of tissue which, after preparation by cutting sections and suitable staining, is examined under the microscope

25. Place the tissue in formalin-saline solution in a container, labelled with the patient's details. The container is sent to the pathology laboratory

26. What are the uses of the following:
   (a) retractors?
   (b) Warwick James' elevators?
   (c) Cryer's elevators?

27. What is meant by an impacted tooth?

28. Name four types of wisdom tooth impaction

29. What pathological conditions may be associated with a partially erupted impacted tooth?

30. What factors help the operator to decide the line of a surgical incision?

31. What is the reason for using curved suture needles in the mouth?

32. Why is strict sterility necessary for minor oral surgical procedures?

33. What is osteomyelitis?

34. When carrying out surgical extractions of lower wisdom teeth, the operator and assistant must take care not to damage a nerve lying close to the inner surface of the mandible. What is this nerve called?

35. What is an oro-antral communication (fistula)?

36. How might an oro-antral communication be caused during dental treatment?

37. What post-operative instructions are given to a patient to help prevent an oro-antral communication?

38. What is an alveolectomy, and what are common reasons why it is used?

39. What is meant by pericoronitis?

26. (a) To retract cheeks, tongue and soft tissues at the site of operation
    (b) Elevation of roots or teeth needing light forces
    (c) Elevation of roots or teeth requiring medium forces

27. One which cannot erupt into the normal position because of obstruction by another tooth or by bone

28. (a) Vertical
    (b) Mesio-angular
    (c) Horizontal
    (d) Disto-angular

29. Pericoronitis, caries, apical abscess

30. (a) Adequate room for access and visibility to the underlying tissues
    (b) Avoidance of important nerves and blood vessels
    (c) A good blood supply to ensure healing

31. In the limited space available a curved needle makes it easier to pass through the tissues

32. Infection introduced into the wound would delay healing, cause the patient discomfort and retard recovery

33. Inflammation of the bone

34. Lingual nerve

35. A connection between the maxillary antrum and the mouth; when this is lined by epithelial tissue it is called an oro-antral fistula

36. The roots of the upper premolars and molars lie immediately below the antrum. Sometimes the roots help to form the floor of the antrum and removal of that tooth creates the opening. Sometimes some of the bone forming the floor of the antrum is extracted with the tooth

37. When the operator considers that the extraction of a tooth may have created a connection, the patient should be advised not to blow his/her nose or to rinse vigorously for a few days

38. The removal of part of the alveolar process i.e. tooth supporting bone
    Used:
    (a) To prepare the mouth for dentures
    (b) To improve the patient's appearance. As an example, a patient with a prominent pre-maxilla may have an alveolectomy when the upper anterior teeth are extracted

39. Inflammation in the soft tissues around the crown of a tooth

40. Why does pericoronitis occur?

41. Why do surgeons and their assistants wear head caps and face masks when operating?

42. Name the instruments commonly used to remove alveolar bone

43. What is the use of a Hunt's syringe?

44. Why are disposable scalpel blades used in surgery?

45. What are the uses of Coupland's chisels?

46. What is blood clotting?

47. When does primary haemorrhage occur?

48. When does reactionary haemorrhage occur?

49. Why does reactionary haemorrhage occur?

50. What can the DA do to help a patient who returns with a bleeding socket? (Assume the absence of the dental surgeon from the practice)

51. When does secondary haemorrhage occur?

52. What is the usual cause of secondary haemorrhage?

53. What is meant by the term 'dental splinting'?

40. It is often associated with partially erupted lower wisdom teeth. Food stagnates under the gum flap and leads to inflammation, which may be acute or chronic

41. To reduce possible contamination of the wound. Face masks are less effective when they become damp with breath

42. Coupland's chisel, mallet and bone chisel, rongeur's bone nibblers, burs, bone files

43. (a) To irrigate and cool burs with a sterile solution during bone removal
(b) To syringe sockets with sterile water or saline solution

44. (a) Blades are blunted in use, a new blade is used for each patient
(b) Reduces the incidence of cross-infection

45. (a) As elevators
(b) Removal of bone

46. Coagulation of blood at the site of a damaged blood vessel

47. Immediately a blood vessel is damaged

48. 1–6 hours after extraction

49. When the vasoconstrictor effect of the local anaesthetic solution wears off there is vasodilatation. The inflammatory response to tissue injury is also occurring. These together can lead to further haemorrhage

50. (a) Check if patient has followed post-operative instructions
(b) Remove excess blood clot with a clean gauze
(c) Roll up gauze swabs to thick finger size and place over socket
(d) Get patient to bite on this pack for at least five minutes
(e) Contact the dental surgeon for advice
(f) Repeat pack procedure if necessary
(g) If bleeding persists call the dental surgeon
(h) Record what has occurred in the patient's notes

51. From the fourth day after extraction and onwards

52. Infection in the wound leading to breakdown of the healing blood vessels

53. Stabilization of loose or damaged teeth or jaw bone using adjacent hard tissues for support

54. When are splints used in dentistry?

55. What types of materials are used to splint teeth after tooth trauma?

56. For a patient with a fractured mandible, what are the common methods of fixation?

57. What are major problems for patients wearing splints?

54. (a) Trauma–to stabilize fractured jaws, loosened teeth
   (b) Oral surgery–in cases where there has been extensive bone loss
       e.g. cysts or following major surgery such as orthognathic
       surgery
   (c) Orthodontics–to retain teeth in their new position
   (d) Periodontics–to stabilize mobile teeth
55. (a) Temporary–lead foil, stainless steel wire
   (b) Longer term–plastic splint
56. (a) With most teeth present–stainless steel wires
   (b) With a few teeth–stainless steel arch bars and wires or silver cap
       splints and connectors
   (c) With no teeth–patient's dentures or Gunning splints which are
       like bite blocks in acrylic, both are stabilized by wiring to bone

57. Appearance, feeding, oral hygiene

Dental materials

Questions

1. What are the uses of zinc oxide and eugenol in dentistry?
2. What are the problems associated with the use of eugenol in the mouth?
3. What are the uses of dental cements in dentistry?
4. Give examples of the forms in which wax is supplied for dental use
5. What basic process is used in the construction of metal crowns and dentures as well as acrylic dentures?
6. What types of material can be used to obtain an accurate fit to edges of impression special trays?
7. State the disadvantage of impression materials which become rigid on setting
8. List the types of 'rigid' impression material
9. What is meant by elastic impression materials?
10. List the types of elastic impression material
11. What are the advantages of elastic impression materials?
12. What are thermoplastic impression materials?

Answers

1. Conservation –temporary filling and cavity lining
   Prosthetics –as a paste for impressions
   Endodontics –as a root sealer
   Periodontics –as a periodontal pack when mixed with cotton wool
   Surgery –mixed with fibres of cotton wool for a socket pack

2. (a) Produces a hot feeling on the mucosa of some patients
   (b) Strong taste which some find unpleasant

3. Conservation –cavity linings, fixing inlays and crowns, and temporary fillings
   Orthodontics –fixing stainless steel bands to teeth
   Oral surgery –fixing splints to teeth

4. Sheet wax –used in denture work and in occlusal registration
   Stick wax –blue for inlay and crown work
   –yellow sticky e.g. used as an impression tray adhesive, temporary fixation of broken items
   Ribbon wax –used in tray modification
   –blocking out unwanted interdental spaces before impression taking
   Impression wax –special impression technique (Applegate)
   Wax patterns –for cast metal denture construction
   Composition –wax is a major constituent

5. The 'lost wax process' in which a wax pattern embedded in a mould is melted away and replaced by hot metal or acrylic dough

6. (a) Greenstick composition
   (b) Mouth curing acrylic e.g. Peripheral Seal

7. The impression cannot be removed from undercut areas except by breaking it

8. Inlay waxes, impression compound, impression plaster, impression paste

9. Impression materials which when slightly deformed will accurately return to their original shape

10. Irreversible hydrocolloids (alginate), reversible hydrocolloids (agar-agar), silicones, polyethers, polysulphide rubbers

11. (a) They can be used in dentate mouths where there are undercut areas
    (b) They do not easily tear or distort

12. Materials which on warming become soft and pliable but become rigid again on cooling

13. Name the most commonly used thermoplastic impression material

14. What material is poured into impressions to produce models of dental arches?

15. Which materials can be used to take impressions of gold inlay cavities?

16. Which materials are commonly used to take final impressions for the following:
    (a) metal partial dentures?
    (b) gold crowns?
    (c) removable orthodontic appliances?
    (d) gum shields?

17. Why is it important to follow the manufacturer's instructions regarding impression materials?

18. How can infection on impressions of a patient's mouth be reduced?

19. How is impression compound prepared for use in taking impressions of an edentulous mouth?

20. When preparing thermoplastic materials what happens if they are made much too hot?

21. What are the dental uses of gutta percha?

22. Articulating paper is used in which procedures?

23. Why is articulating paper used?

24. List the types of 'strips' used in dentistry

13. Impression compound

14. Plaster of Paris (white and relatively soft) or harder materials known as dental stones (coloured and harder)

15. (a) Elastomeric material
    (b) Reversible hydrocolloid
    (c) Brownstick composition in copper ring
    (d) Blue inlay wax (produces an impression which can be cast directly)

16. (a) Alginate, silicones
    (b) Silicones, polyethers, polysulphides
    (c) Alginate
    (d) Alginate, silicones

17. The accuracy of fit of the final work depends upon the quality of the impression. Not following the instructions can result in excessive expansion or contraction, air bubbles, distortion etc.

18. (a) Use of an antiseptic mouthwash prior to impression taking
    (b) More effective is immersion of the impression in an antiseptic for 1 minute then rinsing under running water. Aldehyde 2% solution or sodium hypochlorite 1000 p.p.m. can be used, but rinsing is essential because retained chemical can affect the surface of the impression and damage the skin of any person handling it

19. Place the composition on gauze in a bowl of warm water. When soft it should be moulded by hand and replaced in warm water to ensure that uniform softness is maintained

20. The material becomes sticky and loses its properties

21. Root canal fillings, temporary fillings, soft linings for dentures and splints, testing tooth vitality when warmed

22. (a) After placement of any restoration:
    fillings, crown, bridge and inlay occlusal checks, full and partial denture occlusal checks
    (b) Natural occlusion checks

23. The dye in the paper leaves marks showing where there is heavy or premature occlusion during function

24. (a) Clear and metal matrix strips
    (b) Metal abrasive strips
    (c) Tooth and restoration polishing strips

25. What are the ideal requirements of a temporary filling?

26. Which materials are used in the construction of temporary crowns?

27. A permanent filling material expands and contracts with temperature changes. Why is this necessary?

28. Why should care be taken to exclude as much air as possible from the mix of filling materials?

29. What is the difference between composition and composites?

30. List the uses of composites

31. What is a micro-fine composite?

32. What is a dentine bonding agent?

33. List the uses of glass ionomer cements

34. What is the difference between an etchant and a tooth conditioner?

35. Which materials can be used as fissure sealants?

25. (a) Non-irritant to the dentine and the pulp
   (b) Not easily dislodged from the cavity by the patient
   (c) Easily removed by the operator

26. (a) Crown forms–celluloid, polycarbonate (acrylic), metal (aluminium, stainless steel)
   (b) Alginate as mould of original tooth
   (c) Temporary crown materials–acrylics e.g. Sevriton; resins e.g. Trim, Pro-tem, Scutan
   (d) Filling materials–composites
   (e) Temporary cementation materials–zinc oxide/eugenol type, Temp-bond, zinc cement or polycarboxylate cements

27. To match similar minute changes of the teeth

28. Inclusion of air leads to weakness of the set material

29. Composition is a thermoplastic impression material whereas composites are filling materials

30. As fissure sealants, permanent filling material, tooth facing material, adhesive bridge cement, orthodontic attachment bonding

31. A composite material with very fine particles. A better surface polish can be produced but it wears more easily

32. A resin used as an intermediate layer to aid chemical attachment of restorative material to the dentine

33. As an adhesive lining, luting cement, permanent filling, fissure sealant

34. An etchant contains 30–50% phosphoric acid which decalcifies some of the enamel. A conditioner contains tannic acid or polyacrylic acid and is used to cleanse the surface of the dentine or enamel

35. Composite resin either chemically or light cured, glass ionomer cement

Prosthetics

Questions

1. Give some examples of non-dental prostheses
2. List some reasons for replacing extracted teeth
3. What is a partial denture?
4. Name the materials commonly used as bases for partial dentures
5. What are the likely problems when a partial denture does not fit closely against the adjacent teeth?
6. There are three basic types of partial dentures–what are they?
7. How are partial dentures retained in the mouth?
8. Give the common reasons why patients want partial dentures
9. When visually assessing a patient's mouth prior to making partial dentures what does the operator look for?
10. What is meant by the following:
    (a) a lingual bar?
    (b) an occlusal rest?
    (c) a clasp?
    (d) a skeleton denture?
    (e) a saddle?
11. Why is it advisable to carry out the majority of conservation treatment before taking final impressions for dentures?

Answers

1. False eyes, nose, ear, leg, hand

2. (a) Function
      (i) masticatory efficiency
      (ii) maintenance of remaining dentition
      (iii) prevention of migration of adjacent teeth
   (b) Appearance
   (c) Speech
   (d) Prevention of temporo-mandibular joint problems

3. An artificial replacement for one or more teeth and their supporting structures in an arch, but not all the teeth

4. Acrylic (polymethyl methacrylate), cobalt chrome

5. (a) Food packing occurs and in consequence damage to the gingival margins
   (b) A loose ill-fitting denture

6. (a) Tissue borne, where the denture rests solely on the soft tissues
   (b) Tooth borne, where all the occlusal stress is borne by the teeth
   (c) Tooth/tissue–a combination of the above

7. (a) Friction between natural teeth and denture
   (b) Clasps
   (c) Adhesion (suction) between denture base and mucosa
   (d) Sometimes precision attachments are used

8. Appearance, difficulty in eating

9. (a) Evidence of good oral hygiene
   (b) Good periodontal health
   (c) Low incidence of active caries
   (d) The condition of the tissues covered by any existing denture

10. (a) A metal connection joining two saddle areas of a lower partial denture
    (b) An extension of the denture on to the occlusal surface of a natural tooth to transfer some of the masticatory load of the denture on to that tooth
    (c) A flexible metal extension from a denture to aid retention
    (d) A cast metal partial upper denture designed as a framework rather than a full palatal coverage
    (e) The part of the denture carrying artificial teeth

11. (a) Further extractions may be necessary
    (b) Caries should be under control
    (c) It is easier to make a denture to fit restorations than the other way round

12. Give the contraindications to making partial dentures for patients

13. How do dentures aid plaque retention?

14. Why are patients advised to leave out their dentures at night?

15. How can patients remove plaque from a single natural tooth space?

16. Why might partial dentures be made and fitted before a clearance?

17. Why should particular care be taken with final impressions for a metal denture?

18. Give the most important properties of impression materials for partial dentures

19. List the impression materials suitable for partial dentures

20. What should the DA do with an alginate impression after it has been removed from the mouth?

21. What is the major difference in the care of elastomeric impressions?

22. What will happen if an alginate impression is allowed to get too dry or too wet and what will be the consequences?

23. What should be the temperature of the materials used for mixing alginates?

24. Give the methods by which alginate can be retained in an impression tray

12. (a) High incidence of active dental disease
    (b) Poor oral hygiene
    (c) Uncontrolled epilepsy

13. (a) Preventing natural cleansing of teeth by tongue and saliva
    (b) Clasps, rests etc. are additional plaque retention areas

14. Since 100% oral hygiene is difficult to achieve patients are advised to do this because:
    (a) it enables good cleaning of the natural dentition to be carried out before going to bed
    (b) denture stagnation areas are removed
    (c) micro-organisms in and on the denture can be killed during overnight immersion in a mild antiseptic
    Patients who grind their denture teeth at night also damage the mucosa beneath and so leaving out dentures at night helps to reduce the trauma

15. (a) Using a small toothbrush, possibly an interspace type as well
    (b) Use of dental tape floss or ribbon gauze

16. To help the patient get used to wearing dentures

17. (a) The metal is very hard and difficult to adjust
    (b) The cost of remaking is high

18. (a) Accuracy
    (b) Elasticity without permanent distortion because the impression has to be removed from undercut areas

19. (a) Hydrocolloids e.g. alginate
    (b) Elastomerics e.g. silicones and polyethers (rubber base has a long setting time)

20. (a) Wash off any debris and saliva
    (b) Rinse in antiseptic, wash under running water and then drain
    (c) Carefully wrap it in a damp cloth and seal it in a plastic bag bearing the patient's name. Care must be taken not to distort the impression
    (d) Get it to the laboratory as soon as possible

21. They should not be kept damp

22. It will distort, leading to an inaccurate model, and an ill-fitting denture or appliance

23. Room temperature

24. (a) Tray perforation
    (b) Special adhesive
    (c) Softened sticky wax
    (d) Sticky wax and cotton wool

25. Why is it important that the impression does not become detached from the tray?

26. Ideally an alginate impression should be cast within 20 minutes--why is this?

27. Why are special tray impressions taken?

28. At the partial denture fit appointment, articulating paper may be used–what would this show?

29. What aspects of care of partial dentures should patients understand at the fit appointment?

30. Why should partial dentures be removed before taking part in sports?

31. What items should be laid out for a fit partial denture appointment?

32. What is an overdenture?

33. What special hygiene care do overdenture wearers need to take?

34. What is an immediate denture?

35. What is the major disadvantage of immediate dentures?

36. List the advantages of immediate dentures

37. What in particular is the dental surgeon looking for when examining the mouth before making new full dentures?

38. Which tissues bear the forces of mastication in the natural dentition?

39. Which tissues bear the forces of mastication for full denture wearers?

40. Why should full dentures cover the maximum possible area of mucous membrane?

41. What forces are trying to dislodge dentures?

42. List the impression materials used to obtain impressions of an edentulous mouth

25. Even a slightly detached impression can lead to an inaccurate model

26. Distortion of the impression can begin to occur

27. To ensure greater accuracy of the final model

28. Occlusal high spots or premature contacts

29. (a) Correct insertion and removal of the denture
(b) Denture cleaning instructions
(c) How to store the denture overnight

30. (a) To reduce the chance of denture breakage and possible inhalation of fragments
(b) The denture might come out and be lost or broken

31. Patient's notes, new denture, denture bowl, hand mirror, mouth mirror, handpiece, acrylic trimmer, green abrasive stones, articulating paper, written instructions for patient

32. A denture fitted over the prepared retained roots of teeth

33. Immaculate cleanliness of the face of the retained root

34. A denture bearing one or more teeth, made before the extraction appointment, so that the denture can be inserted as soon as the extraction is completed

35. The large amount of gum shrinkage after extractions, soon leading to a poor fit. Frequent easing may be needed and, ultimately, rebasing or new dentures

36. (a) The patient is never without teeth and therefore is able to eat and has fewer speech problems
(b) It is easier to copy the patient's appearance
(c) Haemostasis
(d) It protects the tooth sockets

37. Retained roots or teeth, swellings–hard or soft, white patches, ulcers

38. Tooth, periodontal ligament and the bone of the socket wall

39. The mucous membrane and bone beneath the denture base

40. To spread the forces of mastication and reduce local pressure

41. (a) Muscles of tongue and cheek
(b) Adhesion of sticky food
(c) For the upper denture–gravity as well

42. Impression composition, plaster of Paris, alginate, zinc oxide–eugenol paste, elastomeric materials

43. During the taking of impressions for a patient
    (a) what is the complication most likely to occur?
    (b) why might this occur?

44. What is a functional impression?

45. How does the operator obtain the greatest accuracy of the flange edges of an impression?

46. Why does the operator ask the patient to move his or her tongue around after seating the loaded lower impression tray?

47. When taking the so-called 'bite', what does the operator wish to show the dental technician?

48. What is meant by freeway space?

49. What needs to be recorded at the 'bite' stage apart from the 'bite'?

50. What is a face bow?

51. Why is there a try-in stage in full denture construction?

52. What does the dental surgeon check at the try-in?

53. What would be the appearance of patients with dentures having:
    (a) too great a vertical dimension
    (b) too little denture support?

54. How may the dentist and the technician make denture teeth look more natural?

55. Why is the posterior edge of an upper denture made to press more firmly into the palatal mucosa than the remainder of the fitting surface?

56. Why might articulating paper be used at the 'fit' appointment?

57. How should dentures be stored when not in the mouth?

43. (i) Retching
(ii) Due to materials touching the back of the tongue or soft palate

44. An impression of the mouth taking account of the position of the tissues during eating, swallowing and speaking

45. By tracing the periphery of the impression tray with a special material such as greenstick composition or one of the mouth setting acrylics

46. To mould the impression material to take account of the movement of the tongue and floor of the mouth during function

47. (a) Length and position of the upper teeth
(b) Vertical distance between the jaws
(c) The naturally retruded position of the mandible
(d) Sometimes the protrusive position of the mandible

48. The space between the teeth of each dental arch when the patient is relaxed. People do not normally keep their teeth clenched together

49. Tooth shade, tooth shape, lip contour

50. An instrument to record the relationship of the maxilla to the temporo-mandibular joint. It is used so that in the laboratory, models of the upper teeth can be placed on an articulator in the same relationship as that of the patient

51. As the teeth are set in wax it allows easy adjustment to correct any errors of teeth and gumwork, or to accommodate changed ideas

52. (a) Appearance of the dentures–arrangement and shade of teeth
(b) Periphery of the wax dentures
(c) Vertical and horizontal relationships of the jaws

53. (a) Stretched skin around the mouth, as if they had a full mouth
(b) Sunken, especially the lips with creasing at mouth corners

54. (a) Selection of suitably shaped and shaded anterior teeth
(b) Slight variation in the setting of individual teeth e.g. producing gaps or slight rotations
(c) Showing the correct amount of tooth when the patient is at rest and when talking
(d) Giving correct support for the lips and cheeks
(e) By incisal grinding to give the appearance of tooth wear

55. To form a vacuum and food seal, called the post-dam line

56. To indicate small errors in occlusion in all movements (high spots)

57. They should be kept moist as the acrylic base may distort if allowed to dry out

58. Why are patients advised to leave out their full dentures at night?

59. Some patients have difficulty in controlling a lower full denture–why is this?

60. Speech may be altered for some patients with new dentures–what are the reasons for this?

61. What advice will be given to patients when new dentures are fitted?

62. What advice should be given about cleaning acrylic dentures?

63. How can plaque on full dentures be demonstrated to patients?

64. Why does calculus collect on dentures?

65. What is a soft lining?

66. How may the fit of a full denture be restored?

67. What is the name applied to the overgrowth of soft tissue associated with a denture flange which is cutting into a patient's mouth?

68. List the materials commonly used to obtain a reline impression

69. What is a tissue conditioner?

70. Why are suction pads not fitted to upper dentures any longer?

58. (a) To rest the soft tissues
    (b) To aid control of infection e.g. prevent denture sore mouth

59. There is little suction and movement of the tongue frequently dislodges the denture

60. Slight changes in artificial tooth position and in the shape of the tongue surface of the denture lead to changes in tongue position which affects speech. Patients quickly adapt to these changes

61. (a) Wearing and cleaning instructions
    (b) Advice about returning if adjustments are needed
    (c) Advice on mouth changes and the need to return for regular examination

62. (a) Over a basin of water–reduces chance of breakage if the denture is dropped
    (b) To use brush of correct size and shape to clean all surfaces
    (c) To use cleaning agent with the brush to remove food debris, grease and plaque
    (d) When using special cleaners to follow the manufacturer's instructions especially about dilution

63. By use of disclosing solution swabbed over the denture

64. Inefficient cleaning

65. A material used on the fitting surface of a denture which remains soft at mouth temperature for some time. It helps to cushion the mucosa from pressure of the denture

66. By making a new denture or by relining or rebasing

67. Denture hyperplasia

68. Zinc oxide–eugenol paste, tissue conditioners and elastomeric impression materials can be used

69. A plastic material which remains soft for a few days during which time the denture bearing tissues can return to their natural condition

70. (a) They do not work
    (b) They can cause perforation of the hard palate and have been known to cause cancer of the hard palate

Instrument and material layouts

Questions

List in order of use the instruments and materials needed for each of the following procedures:

1. Oral hygiene instruction
2. Periodontal assessment
3. Orthodontic diagnosis
4. Taking a blood specimen
5. Administering a local anaesthetic by injection
6. Simple extraction of an upper second premolar under local anaesthesia
7. Repair of oral mucosa by suturing
8. Removal of lower first permanent molar roots
9. Biopsy of soft tissue

Answers

Some optional or alternative items have been included: these are shown in parentheses. The lists would be suitable for most operators but some extra items may be required to suit personal techniques

1. Hand mirror, disclosing agent, cotton wool, tweezers, mouthwash, selection of toothbrushes, floss, wood points, printed instructions

2. Patient records, radiographs, periodontal chart, periodontal probe

3. Patient records, radiographs, orthodontic chart, study models, measuring aids–ruler, dividers, protractor

4. (a) Rubber gloves, plastic apron, yellow plastic waste bag, disposable receiving dish, sharpsafe box
   (b) Tourniquet, antiseptic swab, adhesive tape, 10 ml disposable hypodermic syringe and needle or butterfly, adhesive plaster
   (c) Labelled specimen bottle, two small plastic bags for specimen bottle, infection-risk label if appropriate, laboratory request form

5. Cartridge syringe, suitable needle, local anaesthetic cartridge, with or without vasoconstrictor as prescribed, sterilize the end of the cartridge unless removed directly from sterile pack, warm the cartridge to 20–37°C

6. Local anaesthetic tray, upper extraction forceps–premolars, (Couplands chisel), (gauze bite pack)

7. (a) Local anaesthetic tray
   (b) Cheek retractor, (tongue retractor), suitable suction tip, aspirator, needle holder - Ward or Kilner, (some operators use Spencer Wells artery forceps), toothed tissue forceps, (tweezers)
   (c) Suitable presterilized suture pack or sterile half-circle cutting needle and silk, scissors, sterile swabs or gauze

8. (a) Local anaesthetic tray
   (b) Scalpel and suitable blade, periosteal elevator, flap retractor e.g. Austen's, instruments to remove bone e.g. conventional handpiece and oral surgery burs, (mallet and chisels)
   (c) Irrigating liquid e.g. sterile water or saline, irrigating equipment e.g. 20 ml disposable hypodermic syringe and needle
   (d) Elevators e.g. Warrick James, Cryers, lower root extraction forceps, bone trimming instruments e.g. end- or side-cutting bone nibblers
   (e) Suture kit

9. Local anaesthetic tray, scalpel and suitable blade, formal–saline solution in labelled container with lid, suture kit, histopathology request form

10. Gingivectomy

11. Impressions for study models

12. Taking a bite-wing X-ray film

13. Routine conservation; major equipment already available

14. Two surface amalgam restoration, after completion of the cavity preparation

15. First visit for septic root canal therapy

10. (a) Local anaesthetic tray
   (b) Periodontal probe, college tweezers, pocket measuring forceps
   (c) Suction kit including fine surgical tip
   (d) Gingivectomy knife (electro-surgical cutting equipment)
   (e) Sterile swabs or gauze, fine scissors, scaling instruments
   (f) Materials for a pack e.g. Coe-pack, zinc oxide-eugenol-cotton wool dressing, mixing slab or pad and spatula, petroleum jelly

11. (a) Selection of perforated impression trays plus handles, adhesive, alginate powder, water at room temperature, appropriate measures, mixing bowl and spatula
   (b) Bowl of antiseptic for disinfecting the impressions, labelled plastic bag and damp tissue for temporary storage of the impression, wax sheet to record the occlusion, laboratory ticket

12. (a) Select correct size film, bite-wing film holder or tab attached to film, patient's name on film packet
   (b) Machine, plugged in, brought up to the chair and switched on, exposure timer set
   (c) Protection, lead apron ready

13. (a) Basic tray–mirror, probes–right angled, (sickle), (Briault) college tweezers, suction tip and or saliva ejector
   (b) Preparation–selection of low- and high-speed burs, excavators, (chisels or trimmers)
   (c) Placement–selection of plastic instruments–plugger, flat, carver, burnisher, matrix holder and strip, wedges
   (d) materials–cotton wool rolls, lining, (varnish), amalgamator

14. (a) Conservation tray
   (b) Moisture control e.g. cotton wool rolls, saliva ejector
   (c) Lining calcium hydroxide type, (secondary lining material e.g. zinc cement), mixing pad and spatula
   (d) Filling alloy and mercury in amalgamator, matrix holder and strip, wedges, amalgam carrier, containers for mixed amalgam and for waste amalgam

15. (a) Rubber dam tray, sheet of rubber, rubber dam punch, selection of rubber dam clamps, clamp forceps, dam frame or neck strap, dental floss, lubricant jelly, saliva ejector tip and aspirator. If rubber dam is not being used–saliva ejector tip and aspirator, cotton wool rolls.
   (b) Conservation tray
   (c) Endodontic tray–barbed broach, (smooth broach), set of reamers and files or combination instruments sizes 8–80, paper points, scissors, (engine rotary paste filler), (giromatic handpiece and instruments)
   (d) Root dressing tray – irrigating solution e.g. saline or hypochlorite solution 1000 p.p.m., chemical antiseptic or antibiotic paste, cotton wool pledgets, temporary filling material

16. Taking impressions for a porcelain jacket crown, after preparation stage

17. Fitting a gold crown

18. Taking an occlusal registration for F/F dentures

19. Testing the vitality of a tooth

20. To prepare an anaesthetic machine ready, prior to use, for a general anaesthetic

21. Prepare for an intravenous sedation

16. (a) Gingival retraction cord, astringent solution, scissors, applicator
  (b) Suitable upper and lower impression trays
  (c) Impression material for preparation e.g. elastomer, pad, spatula
  (d) Impression of opposing arch, alginate study model tray set up
  (e) Shade guide
  (f) Laboratory work sheet

17. (a) Laboratory models plus the crown
  (b) Conservation tray, (local anaesthetic tray)
  (c) Handpieces–high and slow-speed, straight and contra-angled, suitable burs, stones and discs etc for any necessary trimming or polishing of the crown
  (d) Thin articulating paper, indicator paste or spray, dental floss
  (e) Saliva ejector, cotton wool rolls, suitable luting material, mixing pad and spatula

18. Laboratory models and bite blocks, laboratory work sheet, denture bowl, Willis bite gauge or steel rule and pencil, (Fox's bite plane), (face bow and wax wafers), wax knife, sheet of pink wax, gas burner and matches, bowl of cold water, shade guide (mould guide)

19. (a) Heat–gutta percha, (flat plastic instrument), gas burner, matches
  (b) Cold–ethyl chloride syringe, cotton wool, college tweezers
  (c) Electrical–electric pulptester, cotton wool roll, conducting agent e.g. prophylaxis paste

20. (a) Check cylinders: oxygen–one full and one in use; nitrous oxide–one full and one in use
    'Full', 'In use', and 'Empty' cylinder notices available.
  (b) 'In use' cylinders turned on and giving a good flow of gas when tested
  (c) Check emergency oxygen working
  (d) Top up vaporizer with volatile agent e.g. halothane, enflurane
  (e) Check that suitable mask and anaesthetic tubes are connected

21. (a) Oxygen machine switched on and tested, emergency kit ready including drugs checked, suction equipment tested
  (b) Tourniquet, skin-sterilizing swab, hypodermic syringe, suitable needle or butterfly, ampoule of sedative drug, water for injection
  (c) Adhesive strips, cotton wool roll, local anaesthetic tray

Short essays

Questions

Pathology, microbiology and sterilization

1. What is inflammation, and what are its signs and symptoms?

2. Briefly relate the signs and symptoms of acute inflammation to what is happening in the tissues

3. What are the major headings under which the causes of disease can be listed? Give examples under each heading

4. How does the body resist infection?

5. How can the number of micro-organisms in a surgery be kept to a minimum?

Answers

Pathology, microbiology and sterilization

1. (a) The body's response to injury (4) may be acute (1) or chronic (1)
   (b) Redness (1), warmth (1), swelling (1), pain (1), loss of function (1)   (11 marks)
2. (a) Redness and warmth–dilatation of blood vessels (1) bringing more blood to the area (1)
   (b) Swelling–due to plasma leaving the capillaries (1) and passing into the tissues (1), the inflammatory exudate. White cells also pass through the vessel walls (1)
   (c) Pain–due to the exudate (1) causing pressure (1) on the nerve endings (1)
   (d) Loss of function–caused by pain (1) and by the swelling (1) leading to restriction (1) of movement   (11 marks)
3. (a) Congenital (3)
       (i) genetic (1) e.g. haemophilia (1)
      (ii) intra-uterine infection (1) e.g. German measles (1)
     (iii) drugs in pregnancy (1) e.g. thalidomide (1)
   (b) Acquired (3)
       (i) living organisms (1)–bacteria, viruses (1)
      (ii) dietary lack (1)–rickets (1)
     (iii) chemicals (1)–poisons (1)
      (iv) physical agents (1)–heat, cold, radiation, trauma (1)   (20 marks)
4. (a) Immunity (2) - natural (1) or acquired (1)
   (b) Body secretions (2) - washing away (1) and antibacterial (1) action e.g. skin oils, sweat, tears, nasal secretion, saliva etc. (2)
   (c) Loss of surface cells (2)
   (d) Respiratory cilia (2)   (14 marks)
5. (a) By regular and thorough cleaning of the whole surgery (2), especially washing with disinfectants (1)
   (b) Maintaining good ventilation (2)
   (c) Wiping down working surfaces (1) and major equipment (1) with antiseptics after each patient (1)
   (d) Sterilizing instruments (4)
   (e) Frequent washing (1) of hands to reduce (1) contamination
   (f) Care with disposal of waste (1) including frequent emptying of bin (1)
   (g) Special precautions (2) with patients in known high infection risk groups (2)   (20 marks)

6. List the time-cycle details for common methods of sterilization used in the dental surgery

7. Give the principles for setting up a surgery for routine conservation for a known inoculation-risk patient

8. Give the principles for clearing a surgery after taking impressions of the mouth for a known inoculation-risk patient

6. Boiling water is not steam sterilization
Steam - autoclave - heating-up time (1) plus holding time 134°C (1) for three minutes (1) plus cooling time (1) adds up to a cycle time of about 20 minutes (1)
Hot oven - heating up time (1) plus holding time one hour (1) at 160°C (1) with the door remaining closed (1) plus cooling time (1) adds up to a cycle time of at least 90 minutes (1)   (11 marks)

7. (a) Surgery – need to decide areas of high and low contamination in the surgery (2). Remove unnecessary items from high contamination zone (2) and cover surfaces (1) and equipment (1) with plastic film (1) to simplify cleaning (1) e.g. handles (1), switches (1), area surrounding working tray (2). If spittoon is to be used then cover area around (1) or provide disposable spit bowl (1)
(b) Waste – double yellow plastic bag 'hung' ready for use (2)
– burn bin for any sharp items (2)
(c) Equipment – contaminate as few items as possible (2) therefore only leave the essentials (1), additions can be made as needed (1). If suction is to be used prepare disposable tubing (1) and tip (1). If interceptor bottle in the system then 1/4 fill with 10000 p.p.m. sodium hypochlorite (2)
Sleeve cords of equipment e.g. low-speed motor and lead (1) with plastic bag or special disposable sleeve (1)
(d) Instruments and materials – sterilizable tray with basic instrument requirements (2)
Pass materials (1) into contamination zone using disposable pad, paper sheet (1) or container (1) when required for use (1)
(e) Protective wear for operator (1) and assistant laid out ready (1) e.g. eye shield (1), mask (1), gown (1), gloves (1)   (40 marks)

8. (a) Protective wear must be worn (4)
(b) Place impressions in fresh 2% glutaraldehyde solution (1) or comparable solution in a container with a sealable lid (1) and marked 'Danger – infection' (1)
(c) Mixing bowl and spatula should not have been contaminated but if so, then sterilize (1)
(d) Autoclave any instruments used, if possible the working tray (2)
(e) Place waste material (1), e.g. tissues, mouthwash cup, in yellow plastic waste bag (1)
(f) Remove protective plastic film (1) from all surfaces and equipment, wipe all surfaces (1) with detergent hypochlorite 1000 p.p.m. (1) but soaking the working tray for 30 minutes (1). Wipe any contaminated area of chair or floor with strong hypochlorite solution (1) or similar solution
(g) Place disposable protective clothing in waste bag (1), seal (1), label 'Danger – infection' (1) and send for incineration (1). Wash hands thoroughly (1)   (22 marks)

Anatomy and physiology

9. Compare and contrast enamel and dentine
10. In simple terms what is the mechanism of breathing?
11. In simple terms what is the mechanism of gaseous exchange in the capillaries?
12. What are the functions of blood?

Anatomy and Physiology

9. Enamel forms the extremely hard (1) covering of the crowns (1) of teeth
Dentine forms the bulk of the tooth (1) within the enamel (1) and the cementum (1) and is softer (1)
Colour – enamel whitish (1), dentine more yellow (1)
Microscopically – enamel made up of prisms (1), dentine of tubules (1)
Composition – enamel 96% calcium salts (1), dentine 70% salts (1)
Sensitivity – enamel is insensitive (1), whereas dentine is sensitive (1)
Regrowth – enamel cannot grow once formed (1). Odontoblasts (1) line the pulpal surface (1) of the dentine and can form new dentine (1)   (18 marks)

10. (a) Inspiration: the rib cage expands (1), the diaphragm descends (1); as the volume of the thorax increases (1), there is a suction pull (1) on the lung tissue so that the lungs expand (1). The air pressure in the lungs is now less (1) than atmospheric pressure and air flows into the lungs (1)
    (b) Expiration: the reverse occurs. The volume of the thorax is decreased (1) forcing air out of the lungs (1).   (9 marks)

11. In the tissues (2) – capillary O_2 concentration is high (1), whereas that in the tissues is low (1); thus O_2 diffuses into the tissues (1). The reverse occurs with CO_2 (1)
In the lungs (2) – CO_2 pressure is low in the alveoli (1) and high in the blood (1); CO_2 diffuses out of the blood into the tissues (1). The reverse occurs with O_2 (1).   (12 marks)

12. (a) Transport (2) of
        (i) gases (1) between lungs and the body cells
        (ii) nourishment (1) to the cells
        (iii) waste products (1) for excretion
        (iv) hormones and enzymes (1) to organs and tissues
    (b) Defence (2) by protection against micro-organisms and their toxins
        (i) white cells (1)
        (ii) antibodies (1)
        (iii) antitoxins (1)
        (iv) wound plugging (1) i.e. blood clotting (1)
    (c) Maintenance of body fluid (2)
    (d) Regulation of body temperature (2)   (17 marks)

13. Describe the neuromuscular events which follow treading, bare-footed, on a pin

14. What are the five main stages in the digestive process?

Instruments, materials and drugs

15. How should surgical scissors be cared for? Give reasons.

16. What types of mouth props are there? Give examples and their uses

17. How is slab impression compound made ready for use?

13. This is a reflex action (2). Pain stimulus (1) to the foot is received by skin receptors (1). The stimulus passes along afferent nerves (1) to the spinal cord (1). Reaction to the stimulus (1) passes along efferent nerves (1) to the leg. A motor response (1) occurs in the muscles (1) of the leg and foot, resulting in the withdrawal (1) of the foot from the pin. Other impulses travel to the brain (1) which lead to controlled, but slightly later reactions (1) e.g. 'Ouch!'

(13 marks)

14. (a) Ingestion (2) – taking in food (1)
(b) Digestion (2) – breakdown of food (1)
(c) Absorption (2) – digested food passes through lining membrane (1)
(d) Assimilation (2) – the food is used by the body cells (1)
(e) Egestion (2) – the expulsion of undigested food (1) and waste products (1)   (16 marks)

Instruments, Materials and Drugs

15. To be used for surgical purposes only (4). After use cleaned (2) to remove blood etc. Check for sharpness (1) and, if necessary, arrange for regrinding (1). If satisfactory, lightly oil (1) the joint, then sterilize (2). Sterilize by dry heat (2), not above 160°C (1) which might spoil the temper (1) of the metal, or by autoclave (2) with a drying cycle (1). Moisture can cause corrosion (1) and bluntness (1) of the blades   (20 marks)

16. (a) Fixed (4) – metal with rubber bite pads (2), or all rubber (2) e.g. Hewitt's (1) or McKesson's (1). Used to keep mouth open (2) during general anaesthesia (1); during a surgical extraction (1) under local analgesia or during prolonged conservation (1)
(b) Spring (2) – e.g. Brunton's (1). Used in conservation (1) and extractions (1) to keep the mouth open (2). Placed in midline (1) and can be swung to the non-working side (1)   (24 marks)
Note – a mouth gag is not a mouth prop

17. Water is heated (1) to the temperature recommended (2) by the manufacturer. A suitable bowl (1) is put out and lined with thin cloth or gauze (1) to prevent the composition sticking (1) to the bowl. The warm water is placed in the bowl (1) plus the appropriate amount of slab composition (1). These are allowed to soften (1), are moulded (1) in the hands, replaced in the water to resoften and then remoulded (1). The composition should then be evenly soft (1) and should be left in the water, maintained at the correct temperature (1) prior to loading the impression tray.   (13 marks)

18. How should drugs used in dentistry be cared for?

19. There are four main routes of administration of drugs used in connection with dentistry. Name them, giving one example of each

20. Many types of syringes are found in the dental surgery. List them and state how they should be dealt with after use

18. (a) Drugs must be kept in containers with secure lids (1), preferably 'child-proof' (1).
   (b) All containers must be properly labelled (4). Labels must carry information giving the name of the contents (2) and the strength of the contents (2). Adding the date of purchase and/or expiry (1) to each container label should prevent out of date stock being used (1). Contents of unlabelled containers (1) should be safely discarded (2)
   (c) Stocks should be kept tidy (1); this will reduce overstocking (1)
   (d) Storage – all drugs must be kept in a safe place (1), out of easy reach of unauthorized persons (1) and preferably in a lockable cupboard (1). Storage should be in cool dry (1) conditions unless the manufacturer advises otherwise (1).
   (e) Drugs of addiction (2) and drugs acting on the central nervous system (2) must be kept in a locked cupboard (2)
   (f) Maintain a record of purchase (1) and use (1) of drugs. This will also be useful in stock control (1). All poisons must be clearly labelled poison (2)   (33 marks)

19. (a) Oral (2) either in tablet or capsule form (1) or in liquids (1)
   (b) Injection (2) e.g. intramuscular (1) – antibiotics (1)
                      intravenous (1) – sedation or anaesthesia (1)
                      submucous (1) or block dental analgesia (1)
   (c) Topical (2) via mucous membrane e.g. analgesic ointment (1)
   (d) Inhalation (2) e.g. anaesthetic gases (1)
                      decongestants for sinusitis (1)   (19 marks)

20. (a) Equipment – unit 3-in-1 syringe (2). At least wipe nozzle (1), handle (1), control switches (1) and syringe holder on unit (1) with an antiseptic agent (2). Ideally the nozzle is sterilized (2) between patients (2), or immersed in a strong antiseptic solution for 30 minutes (2) and then rinsed thoroughly (1) before use on another patient. This must be carried out at the end of each session (2) and if used for an inoculation-risk patient. (3)
   (b) Cartridge types – barrel (2) and breech (2) loading, aspirating (1) and non-aspirating (1), intra-ligamentary (2), needle (1) and cartridge (1) should be carefully (1) discarded into a Sharp's box (2). Syringe physically cleaned (1), then sterilized (2)
   (c) Disposable – hypodermic (2) (many sizes (1) and impression (2) Hypodermic must be carefully (1) discarded together with the needle (1) into a Sharp's box (2). As nozzle of impression syringe may perforate waste bags, place it in a Sharp's box (1)
   (d) Non-disposable – hypodermic (1), impression (1), Hunt's (1) and chip (1). The hypodermic needle (1) and impression tip (1) are placed in the Sharp's box . In all types they are dismantled (1), cleaned (1), sterilized (2) and then reassembled (1)
                                                    (56 marks)

21. How can a clean, dry working site be maintained for all types of dental treatment?

22. What are the usual errors in mixing alginate impression materials and what are the results of these errors?

21. (a) A pre-requisite is that the patient has good oral hygiene (1) and cleans his/her mouth before (1) the appointment. A further aid to a clean site is to use the 3-in-1 syringe (1) and suction (1) immediately before (1) treatment

   (b) Cleaning achieved by use of irrigating solution (2) examples :
     (i) conservation (1) – turbine spray (1), 3-in-1 syringe (1)
     (ii) endodontics (1) – saline in hypodermic syringe (1), local anaesthetic solution (1)
     (iii) scaling (1) – 3-in-1 (1), ultrasonic water (1)
     (iv) surgery (1) – 3-in-1 prior to cutting (1), sterile solutions (1) in hypodermic syringe (1) or from a drip system (1)

   (c) Control of fluids (1) e.g. saliva (1), blood (1) and irrigating solutions (1) is needed

   (d) Control achieved by :
     (i) position (1) – body and head position can help (2)
     (ii) instruments (1) – suitable size suction tip, saliva ejector (3)
     (iii) materials (1) – cotton wool rolls, dry pads, rubber dam (3)
     (iv) equipment (1) – 3-in-1 or chip syringe (2)
     (v) irrigants (1) – control of volume to give clean site but easy drying (2)
     (vi) drugs (1) – vasoconstrictor to control bleeding – rare use of drugs to control saliva flow (2)   (45 marks)

22. (a) Powder container not shaken (2) to mix contents (1), heavier particles (1) containing retarder (1) stay at the bottom (1)
     Result –
     (i) Faster set with powder from top of container (1)
     (ii) Slow set with last of contents (1)
     (iii) Dense powder leading to stiff mix (1)

   (b) Too much powder (2), caused by tapping the powder scoop (1)
Result – stiff mix (1), difficult for operator to insert (1), probable distortion (1) of soft tissues and inaccuracy of the impression (1)

   (c) Water too warm (2)
Result – material sets quickly (1), difficult, perhaps impossible, to insert (1), possible need to retake impression (1)

   (d) Insufficient spatulation (2)
Result – dry powder (1) in patches – inaccurate impression (1); air bubbles (1) not removed – inaccuracy (1) and if large bubbles possible weakness and tearing of impression (1)
       (28 marks)

23. What is the acid-etch system and how does it help in retention?

24. Briefly state the properties of the ideal filling material.

Hazards

25. What is the role of the DA in preventing and dealing with a fire at a dental surgery?

23. It is a method of physically bonding composite (1) materials to enamel (1). A weak acid solution (1) is applied to the tooth, cleansing (1) the enamel surface and removing (1) small amounts of the enamel prisms (1) called etching (1), thus creating hundreds of short tubular deficiencies (1) in the enamel surface (1). The composite flows (1) into these deficiencies and when set provides hundreds of anchorage tags (1) helping to retain (1) the restoration.

(12 marks)

24. (a) Should not affect the health of the patient (2) or the oral tissues (2)
   (b) Should be able to withstand acid foods etc (1)
   (c) Should not react with other materials (2) in the oral environment to produce galvanic (1) or other unwanted effects (1)
   (d) Should expand and contract (2) with temperature changes (1) in a similar manner to tooth tissues (1)
   (e) Should be able to withstand masticatory forces (2)
   (f) Should have a pleasing appearance (1)
   (g) Should have sufficient working time (1) and set (1) within a reasonable time
   (h) Should have minimum corrosion (1)   (19 marks)

Hazards

25. Prevention – Careful use of electrical equipment (1)
                    Report any faults immediately (1)
                    Ensure safe use of naked flames, matches, gas burners (2)
                    Correct storage of inflammable materials (1)
                    Switch off electrical and gas equipment when not in use (1) and at mains overnight (1)
   Safety – Ensure corridors and fire exits are never obstructed (3)
            Knowledge of fire drill (1)
   Fire – Whereabouts of firefighting equipment (1)
          If a fire, try to stop at source (1)
          Raise the alarm including 999 call (1)
          Evacuate the premises (1), making sure no one (1) is left in any room and closing (1) each door
          Check those leaving against appointment book (1), clearly marking (1)
          If possible switch off main gas and electricity (1)

(20 marks)

26. After a needle-stick injury from an instrument used on any patient, what procedure should be followed?

27. How can the DA avoid mercury contamination, and what precautions can be taken when using amalgam for a restoration?

28. How should spillage of mercury be dealt with?

26. (a) First aid Wash under running water (2), squeeze to make wound bleed (1), wash with antiseptic (1)

Apply antiseptic cover (1) with dressing then wear rubber glove or waterproof fingerstall (2)

(b) Report accident to your employer (1) who should:

(c) Recheck medical history (1) – whether patient is in a risk group (1) e.g. hepatitis B (1), HIV (1).

If yes, then urgent (1) hospital treatment needs to be arranged (1), taking patient details (1), including name and address of patient's G.P. (1)

If no, your employer will decide whether 'yes' procedure should still be followed (1)

In any case, if you are unsure consult your own GP (1). You might develop a simple wound abscess or feel unwell with raised temperature (1)   (19 marks)

27. (a) Not to spill mercury (1)

(b) Keep mercury (1) and waste amalgam (1) in a sealed container (1) under water or special solution (1)

(c) Not to wear open-toed shoes (1)

(d) Not to handle mercury (1) or mixed amalgam (1)

(e) Ensure no amalgam fragments go into dry-heat sterilizer (1)

(f) Make sure room is well ventilated (1)

(g) Keep amalgamator in a enclosed container (1)

(h) Stand amalgamator on foil-lined tray to collect any droplets (2)

(i) Do not handle waste amalgam in waste traps (1)

(j) Wash hands after using amalgam (1) or mercury (1) (16 marks)

28. (a) Arrange maximum ventilation (2)

(b) Inform the Dental Surgeon (3)

(c) Wearing rubber gloves (2) and a face mask (2)

   (i) carefully collect obvious mercury into a suitable container (2)

   (ii) to prevent globules running, spread dry sand or flowers of sulphur (2) over the area and then sweep (2) the area taking special care to empty any surface cracks (2)

   do not use vacuum cleaner (1) or dental suction machines (1)

(c) All spilt mercury to be stored in a closed container under water (2)

(d) Careful disposal of cleaning equipment, gloves and mask (1)

(22 marks)

Dental disease

29. What clinical, epidemiological and experimental evidence is available to associate refined carbohydrate with dental caries?
30. What advice can be given to children regarding prevention of dental disease?
31. What are the consequences of a deepening periodontal pocket?

Dental Disease

29. (a) Clinical:
     (i) labial caries (2) of deciduous teeth where comforters (1) containing concentrated syrups (1) and fruit juices (1) have been used a lot
     (ii) sudden increase (2) in number of new cavities (1) in older patients (2) if the amount of sweet eating (1) is greatly increased
   (b) Epidemiological:
     (i) lack of caries in primitive peoples (2) until Western civilization reaches them, and they eat a 'modern' diet (1)
     (ii) fall of caries (2) incidence during the Second World War when there was sugar rationing (1)
   (c) Experimental:
   Vipeholme study (2). This showed the greatest increase (2) in caries with frequent between meals (1) consumption of sugar (1) in sticky form. This effect was reversed (2) when patients returned (1) to a basic diet unsupplemented (1) by sugar   (27 marks)

30. (a) Diet (2)
     (i) restrict (1) between meals snacks (1) and drinks (1)
     (ii) sweets (1) should be eaten after one meal (1) on some days (1). Try to avoid sticky sweets (1)
     (iii) eat a balanced diet (1), avoid excess sugar and carbohydrate (2), restrict intake of citrus fruit and juices (1) as the sweetness masks the damaging acidity (1)
   (b) Oral hygiene (2)
     (i) when – clean after meals or at least rinse (2) and clean before bed (2)
     (ii) how – using mini-scrub or roll technique (2), whichever works best for the patient (1); use a fluoride toothpaste (1)
     (iii) where – all teeth (1), especially remembering the last molars (1)   (26 marks)

31. Increasing difficulty in cleansing the pocket (1), therefore more plaque (2) and more calculus (2). Tissue reaction to the toxins (1) of plaque leads to increasing inflammation of the soft tissues and bone (1). More alveolar bone is resorbed (2) and the tooth becomes loose (2). The tooth may tilt (1) and there is eventual loss of the tooth (2)
                    (14 marks)

32. Name the types of calculus. What are the differences between them?

33. Patients sometimes state that a badly decayed tooth ached severely for a day or so and then suddenly the pain disappeared. What is the usual explanation for this?

34. How may caries become arrested?

35. There are two main processes in dental caries. Name each and state briefly what occurs in each

36. Why is it important to clean the teeth properly after the last food and drink at night?

32. (a) Supragingival (2)
  (i) affects mainly the lower incisors (1) and upper molars (1)
  (ii) colour yellowish (1)
  (iii) site above gum level (1)
  (iv) consistency chalky (1), not too difficult to remove (1)
(b) Subgingival (2)
  (i) affects any teeth (2), often found lingual to lower molars (1)
  (ii) colour dark brown to black (1)
  (iii) site below gum in the gingival crevice (1)
  (iv) consistency hard (1) and tenacious (1)   (17 marks)

33. This answer must relate to the process of acute inflammation. The pulp is infected (2) and inflamed (2) so there is an increased blood supply (2) to the area and formation of inflammatory exudate (2). As there cannot (1) be any swelling within the hard-walled pulp chamber (1), the pressure increases (1) stimulating nerve endings (1) of the pulp and causing pain. If this pressure is relieved (2), i.e. drainage into the mouth (1) or through the apex into the softer tissues (1) in the periapical area, there will be relief of pain (2)
                                                                            (18 marks)

34. (a) Naturally (2)
  (i) the very early enamel caries lesion can be remineralized (2) following avoidance of demineralizing foods (1) e.g. fruit juices (1), and by the patient using remineralizing solutions, e.g. fluoride mouthwashes (1), fluoride toothpaste (1), mineral salts in the diet and saliva (1)
  (ii) by the tooth substance crumbling away (1) to produce a self-cleansing surface (1)
(b) Artificially (2)
  (i) painting the affected area with topical fluoride (1)
  (ii) the operator removing (1) enamel to produce a self-cleansing area (1) or by cavity preparation (2) and filling (2)
                                                                            (20 marks)

35. (a) Decalcification (2). Acids (1) are produced by the action of bacteria on substrate (1), mainly refined sugars. These acids (1) demineralize or break down (1) calcium salts (1) in the tooth substance. This is the enamel caries process (1)
(b) Proteolysis (2). Certain bacteria (1), present in the mouth, digest (1) the organic content (1) of the tooth. Dentine caries involves both decalcification (1) and proteolysis (1) which are progressing simultaneously (1)   (16 marks)

36. So that minimal plaque (2) is left on the teeth at night. While we are asleep there are minimal movements of the tongue (2) and very little saliva (2) is produced. Plaque therefore remains undisturbed (2) and leads to prolonged attack (2) on dental tissues   (10 marks)

Restorative dentistry

37. How may the DA assist the operator when a change of root canal dressing is being carried out?

38. How can the DA be helpful at the chairside during dental treatment of children?

39. In terms understandable to the average patient, describe the procedure for crowning a molar tooth

Restorative Dentistry

37. (a) By a complete layout (2) of patient's records (1) including radiographs (1), necessary instruments (1) and materials (1)
   (b) Assisting in protection of the pharynx (2) by:
       (i) attaching parachute chain to root canal files etc. (1)
       (ii) careful use of suction tip (1)
       (iii) assisting in application of a rubber dam (1)
   (c) By anticipation (2) in passing of instruments (1) and having materials ready (1) for use
   (d) By taking over (2) some actions from the operator e.g. setting the length of root canal instruments (1) or wetting a paper point in antiseptic (1)   (19 marks)

38. (a) By having necessary instruments (2) and materials (2) available but not on display (1)
   (b) Helping to make sure that the patient is seen on time (2)
   (c) If opportune, by showing the child how the equipment works (1)
   (d) Explaining in suitable language (1) the treatment procedures (1)
   (e) Playing a supporting role to the operator (1)
   (f) Stressing importance of oral hygiene to the child (1) (12 marks)

39. At the first treatment visit (1) usually a local anaesthetic is necessary (1)
   (a) About 1 mm or 1/16 inch (1) of the tooth (1) or filling (1) is removed from all over the crown (1) of the tooth. This gives enough space (1) for the metal (1) of the new crown
   (b) Impressions (1) are taken to get models of the shaped tooth (2) and all other teeth (2), as the technician needs to know how all the teeth meet together (1)
   (c) A temporary crown is made (2) and fitted to protect the tooth (1) and prevent it changing position (1) while the permanent crown is being made. The next appointment is usually a week later (1)
   (d) The technician makes each crown specially for each tooth (1)
   At the second visit (1):
   (e) The temporary crown is removed (1), the gold crown (1) is placed on the tooth and checked for fit (2) and that the teeth meet correctly (2)
   (f) The crown is then permanently cemented (2)   (29 marks)

40. List the surgery stages in the construction of an all-metal bridge

Anaesthesia, first aid and minor oral surgery

41. Local anaesthesia has several advantages over general anaesthesia. State some of these advantages

42. What is the mechanism by which general anaesthetics take effect?

43. What are the duties of the DA during a general anaesthetic?

40. First visit: – assessment (2) – clinical, radiographic, study impressions (3)

Later visit:

(a) Preparation for temporary bridge (1)

(b) Preparation of abutment teeth (1)

(c) Impression taking (1)

(d) Recording of occlusion (1)

(e) Shade taking (1) if needed

(f) Making temporary bridge (1)

(g) Cementing temporary bridge (1)

Next visit:

(a) Removal of temporary bridge (1)

(b) Try in and if necessary make adjustment (1)

(c) Cementation of permanent bridge (1)

(d) Final check of margins and occlusion (1)   (16 marks)

Anaesthesia, First Aid and Minor Oral Surgery

41. (a) Relatively easy to administer (3)

(b) Simpler equipment (1)

(c) Can be used on most patients, some of whom might be unfit for general anaesthesia (3)

(d) Initial control of haemorrhage in surgical cases (2) if solution containing vasoconstrictor is used adjacent to site of surgery

(e) Patient co-operation throughout procedures (2)

(f) No time constraints (1)

(g) Less risk to the patient (2)   (14 marks)

42. The anaesthetic drugs work on the brain (3) but are administered at some remote point (3) e.g. lungs (1) or vein (1) in the hand. A state of unconsciousness (1) is induced and impulses reaching the brain (1) are not felt (1)   (11 marks)

43. (a) Anticipation of needs (2) of the operator or the anaesthetist, depending upon who is being assisted

(b) Passing instruments and materials (2) as required

(c) Keeping operating field clear (2) by careful retraction (1) and good suction (1)

(d) Assisting in monitoring (2) patient's respiration and pulse

(e) Acting as chaperone (2)

(f) Forming part of the surgery team (1)   (13 marks)

44. What are the duties of the DA during a patient's recovery from a general anaesthetic?

45. Describe how mouth-to-mouth resuscitation should be carried out. How can this technique be varied in the surgery?

46. Describe how the chest compression technique (external cardiac massage) should be carried out on an adult. Briefly explain the technique

44. (a) Supporting the patient's head to maintain the airway (3) and to prevent injury to the patient (3)

(b) Monitor respiration (2) and pulse (2) calling the anaesthetist's attention (1) if any variations from normal (1) occur

(c) Use of suction (1) to remove blood (1) and saliva (1) from the mouth and if bleeding persists (1) report it to the dentist (1)

(d) Ensure that, if the patient vomits, none is inhaled (3) (20 marks)

45. (a) The person should be laid on his or her back (2) on a firm surface (2)

(b) Any possible airway obstruction (2) must be removed e.g. foreign body (1) such as denture, or constriction such as tight collar (1)

(c) Extend the person's neck and insert a neck roll (3)

(d) Pinch the nostrils (2)

(e) Place your mouth over the person's mouth (2) ensuring a seal (1)

(f) Blow into the the person's mouth checking that the chest rises (3). If no chest movement then find cause of obstruction (2)

(g) Maintain a rate of at least ten breaths per minute (1) (22 marks)

In the surgery:

(a) After clearing the patient's airway (2) insert an oral airway (2)

(b) Cover the nose and mouth with a close-fitting (1) facemask (2) connected to the oxygen supply (2)

(c) Extend patient's neck and insert neck rest (3)

(d) Inflate lungs with oxygen (2) by squeezing respiratory bag (2)

(e) In all cases help should be summoned (1) and an attempt made to decide the cause of the condition (1) (18 marks)

46. (a) The person should be laid on the floor (2); this is an easier working position (1). Kneel beside the person (1)

(b) The heels of the hands (1) are placed on top of each other (1) over the lower half (1) of the person's sternum (1)

(c) The sternum should then be depressed about 5 cm (1) by applying your full weight. Repeat this once per second (1)

(d) Depressing the sternum will squeeze the heart against the spine (2) forcing blood into the circulatory system (2) (14 marks)

47. How should fainting be treated? Give reasons for each action

48. Briefly list the duties of a DA before, during and after any minor oral surgery procedure

47. (a) Lay the person flat (1), if not already so, or preferably place him or her in the tonsillar position (2). Putting the head between the knees may compress the inferior vena cava, and in fact reduce the blood flow from the legs.

Ideally the legs should be raised above the level of the heart and brain (1) to ensure the blood supply to the brain (1)

(b) Remove any possible airway obstruction (2) e.g. denture, tight collar

(c) If necessary administer oxygen (1)

(d) As the person recovers, reassure (1), but keep flat (1)

(e) As the person's colour returns, raise slowly (1), but lower again if signs of fainting recur (1)

(f) Give the person a glucose drink (1) to raise the blood sugar level (1) which is sometimes low in those who faint   (14 marks)

48. (a) Before:
  (i) Get out patient's notes (1) and radiographs (1)
  (ii) Sterilize (2) all necessary instruments and swab down working surfaces (1) and equipment (1) with antiseptic in spirit (1)
  (iii) Wash hands (1), lay out instruments on a sterile tray (2) using 'non-touch' technique (2), cover tray with sterile cover (1)
  (iv) Get correct patient (1) ready and comfortably seated in the chair (1)

(b) During:
  (i) After scrubbing hands (1) and putting on gloves (1) be prepared to pass instruments (1), retract tissues (1), irrigate (1) and use suction (1) as required.
  (ii) Anticipate (2) the surgeon's requirements
  (iii) Monitor (2) and if necessary, reassure (1) the patient

(c) After:
  (i) Make sure the patient is cleaned up (1) and fit enough (2) to leave the surgery
  (ii) Make sure patient understands post-operative instructions (2)
  (iii) Clean (1) and sterilize (2) all instruments
  (iv) Clean all the working surfaces (1) and attend to the sucker (1)

(36 marks)

Multiple choice

Questions

One or more answers to each question can be correct.

General

1. What is the name for a collection of similar cells grouped together with a special function?
   - (a) organism
   - (b) organ
   - (c) gland
   - (d) tissue
   - (e) system

2. Which component of the blood is responsible for transporting oxygen?
   - (a) red cells
   - (b) white cells
   - (c) plasma
   - (d) phagocytes
   - (e) platelets

3. Where does digestion of starch begin?
   - (a) mouth
   - (b) oesophagus
   - (c) stomach
   - (d) duodenum
   - (e) ileum

4. The normal adult resting rate of respiration is
   - (a) 48
   - (b) 98
   - (c) 72
   - (d) 15
   - (e) 37

5. The normal resting adult pulse rate is
   - (a) 37
   - (b) 16
   - (c) 70
   - (d) 98
   - (e) 104

6. A scald is caused by
   - (a) wet heat
   - (b) dry heat
   - (c) both
   - (d) neither

7. When does secondary haemorrhage occur?
   - (a) immediately a tooth is extracted
   - (b) about 4 hours after extraction
   - (c) if the patient over-exercises
   - (d) when the local anaesthetic wears off
   - (e) if the socket becomes infected

8. After a needlestick injury the most important action is to
   (a) record the event in   (d) inform environmental health
       the accident book   department
   (b) go to the hospital   (e) none of these
   (c) bandage the wound

9. Nitrous oxide is a hazard to female staff in the surgery because
   (a) it causes nausea   (d) they may accidentally inhale it
   (b) they may get sleepy   (e) of possible spontaneous abortion
   (c) it may damage the liver

10. Goggles are worn by the DA during conservation to protect
    against
    (a) oil mist   (d) mercury vapour
    (b) droplet infection   (e) tooth debris
    (c) turbine exhaust

11. What is the best way to dispose of waste amalgam?
    (a) in a sealed container (d) under fluid in a sealed container
    (b) in the waste bin   (e) give to scrap merchant
    (c) wash down the sink

12. Which instruments need regular sharpening?
    (a) excavators   (d) scalers
    (b) carvers   (e) burs
    (c) elevators

13. A prescription for sedative tablets can
    (a) be written and signed by a qualified DA
    (b) have the patient's name and address only written by a DA
    (c) be written by a DA and signed by a dental surgeon
    (d) only be written and signed by a dental surgeon

14. An analgesic drug is one which
    (a) prevents infection   (c) prevents blood clotting
    (b) kills pain   (d) anaesthetizes a patient

15. The disadvantages of aspirin as an analgesic are
    (a) the patient has to starve before taking aspirin
    (b) it is too weak for dental pain
    (c) it does not affect pulpitis
    (d) it can cause gastric upsets

16. Intravenous sedation drugs should be stored
    (a) in a refrigerator   (c) upright in a drawer
    (b) out of reach of children(d) in a locked cupboard

17. Responsibility for sedative drugs in dental practice rests with
    whom?
    (a) the dental surgeon   (c) the senior dental assistant
    (b) any dental assistant

18. Fluoride is added to domestic water supplies to produce a concentration very close to
    (a) 100 parts per million   (c) 4 parts per million
    (b) 10 parts per million   (d) 1 part per million

19. Which organ can be irreparably damaged by rheumatic fever?
    (a) the tongue   (d) the heart
    (b) the liver   (e) the spleen
    (c) the spine

20. Subgingival calculus is always a feature of gingivitis.
    (a) true
    (b) false

21. The most commonly occurring disease of humans is
    (a) heart disease   (d) skin disease
    (b) cancer   (e) arthritis
    (c) gum disease

22. Calculus is usually formed
    (a) in saliva   (c) from saliva
    (b) by water   (d) by the gingival crevice

23. Bleeding gums are a symptom of
    (a) ill health   (d) poor brushing
    (b) soft foods   (e) gingivitis
    (c) caries

24. The main dental use of soft wood points is
    (a) as a mouth prop
    (b) to contour restorations
    (c) to remove interdental plaque
    (d) to remove the interdental papillae

25. Dental floss prevents
    (a) caries
    (b) periodontal disease.
    True or false?

26. The effect on the gingiva of retained plaque is
    (a) formation of calculus
    (b) mouth ulceration
    (c) dental caries
    (d) gingivitis

27. The primary use of dental floss is to
    (a) remove food
    (b) remove excess gingiva
    (c) massage the gingiva
    (d) clean the interproximal surfaces

28. Periodontitis is
  (a) inflammation of the pulp
  (b) dental caries
  (c) inflammation of the periodontal ligament
  (d) calculus
  (e) inflammation of the gingiva

29. Occlusal registration means
  (a) the occlusal surface of the lower wisdom teeth
  (b) the bite stage in prosthetics
  (c) an anterior occlusal radiograph
  (d) the charting of occlusal cavities
  (e) the construction of an obturator

Oral Anatomy

30. A foramen is
  (a) a prominent part of a bone
  (b) a hole in a bone
  (c) a natural opening in a bone for the passage of nerves and vessels
  (d) a groove in the tooth enamel

31. Immediately posterior to the hard palate is the
  (a) tongue   (d) larynx
  (b) soft palate   (e) uvula
  (c) pharynx

32. The mental foramen is situated in
  (a) temporal bone   (d) sulcus
  (b) hard palate   (e) soft palate
  (c) mandible

33. The cranial nerve supplying the teeth and jaws is
  (a) III   (b) IV   (c) V   (d) VII   (e) IX

34. A sensory nerve is one which carries stimuli
  (a) from the peripheral tissues
  (b) to the peripheral tissues
  (c) to the muscles

35. Ophthalmic, maxillary, mandibular are divisions of which cranial nerve?
  (a) I   (b) II   (c) VII   (d) III   (e) V

36. The nerve to the upper jaw contains fibres which are
  (a) sensory   (b) motor   (c) sensory and motor

37. The mandibular nerve is
(a) sensory   (b) motor   (c) sensory and motor

38. Removed from the tooth a healthy pulp looks like
(a) red tape   (c) pink thread
(b) white tape   (d) black thread

39. Name the folds of tissue which attach the gum to the lips in the mid-line.
(a) Mandibular frenum   (d) Buccal frenum
(b) Maxillary flange   (e) Labial frenae
(c) Lingual frenum

40. The tongue is mainly composed of
(a) bone and muscle   (c) adipose tissue
(b) gristle and muscle   (d) muscle fibres

41. Enamel is produced by
(a) Schwann cells   (d) lacunae
(b) osteocytes   (e) ameloblasts
(c) odontoblasts

42. Select from List I the word most suitable to each phrase in List II.
List I
(a) osteoblasts   (e) occlusal
(b) fissures   (f) palatal
(c) contact points   (g) odontoblasts
(d) incise   (h) tear
List II
(1) The prime function of the incisor teeth is to .....
(2) The prime function of the canine teeth is to .....
(3) The cells which form dentine are called .....
(4) Between the cusps of the posterior teeth lie the .....
(5) The cuspal surface of a molar tooth is called the ..... surface

43. Select from List I the word most suitable to each phrase in List II.
List I
(a) amelodental   (f) amelocemental
(b) gingivitis   (g) periodontitis
(c) apex   (h) grind
(d) incisal edge   (i) periodontal
(e) cusp   (j) pericoronitis
List II
(1) The prime function of posterior teeth is to .....
(2) Inflammation around the crown of an erupting tooth is called
.....
(3) The tip of a tooth root is called the .....
(4) The visible line between the crown and the root is called the
..... junction
(5) The biting part of an incisor tooth is the .....

44. The components of dentine are
(a) calcium salts only
(b) calcium salts and some living cytoplasm
(c) calcium salts and blood vessels
(d) calcium salts and hollow tubules
(e) nerve endings and calcium salts

45. Match the words in List I with the conditions in List II
List I
(a) Crown   (f) Occlusal
(b) Mesial   (g) Absorption
(c) Resorption   (h) Lingual
(d) Root   (i) Impaction
(e) Distal   (j) Buccal
List II
(1) Obstruction to the eruption of a tooth
(2) Shortening of the root of a deciduous tooth before natural loss
(3) The parts of a tooth
(4) The surfaces of a tooth

46. Edentulous persons are those
(a) with all their teeth   (c) with no natural teeth
(b) with no teeth   (d) who are unable to eat

47. The tooth is held in its socket by
(a) cementum   (c) periodontal ligament
(b) bone   (d) the gum

48. The maximum number of teeth usually found in the mouth of the human adult is
(a) 20   (b) 28   (c) 24   (d) 32   (e) 36

49. When a tooth erupts
(a) the root is fully formed   (d) the root canal is open
(b) the root is partly formed   (e) no cementum has formed
(c) the root canal is closed

50. The teeth which erupt distal to the deciduous second molars are
(a) deciduous   (b) permanent

51. The roots of permanent teeth are completely formed
(a) when they erupt
(b) six months after eruption
(c) about one year after eruption
(d) about two years after eruption
(e) about three years after eruption

52. What is the usual number of teeth found in the mouth of a four year old child?
(a) 16   (b) 20   (c) 24   (d) 32   (e) 22

53. Which permanent teeth do not have deciduous predecessors?
    (a) molars
    (b) premolars
    (c) canines
    (d) incisors

54. What is the usual sequence of eruption of deciduous teeth?
    (a) a b c d e
    (b) a c b d e
    (c) a b d c e
    (d) a b c e d
    (e) a c b e d

55. Loss of the deciduous dentition is usually completed by the age of
    (a) about 6 years
    (b) about 12 years
    (c) about 8 years
    (d) about 18 years

56. Incisor teeth are those which are
    (a) chisel-shaped cutting teeth
    (b) sharp tearing teeth
    (c) large grinding teeth
    (d) ridged crushing teeth
    (e) pointed flesh-shearing teeth

57. Taste buds are found mainly on the
    (a) tongue
    (b) cheek
    (c) soft palate
    (d) hard palate
    (e) lips

58. The periodontal ligament is composed of
    (a) gingival tissue
    (b) a sheath one cell thick
    (c) elastic fibres only
    (d) fibres, nerves and vessels

59. A diastema is
    (a) an unerupted tooth
    (b) a supernumerary tooth
    (c) a type of orthodontic appliance
    (d) the surgical removal of a buried root
    (e) a wide space between two adjacent teeth

60. What is the name given to the fold of tissue attached to the floor of the mouth between the openings of the submandibular glands?
    (a) labial frenum
    (b) buccal frenum
    (c) mandibular frenum
    (d) palatal frenum
    (e) lingual frenum

61. The gingiva include the
    (a) soft lining of all the mouth
    (b) tissue covering the alveolar bone
    (c) tissue covering the roof of the mouth
    (d) tissue covering the tongue

62. Immediately after eruption the enamel
    (a) continues to calcify
    (b) starts to harden
    (c) changes very little
    (d) continues to form

63. A normal healthy tongue should be
    (a) smooth and shiny
    (b) furred and grey
    (c) white and smooth
    (d) red and shiny
    (e) pink and roughened

64. A lingual flange is
    (a) a growth on the tongue
    (b) a tongue retractor
    (c) part of a molar tooth
    (d) part of a lower denture

Microbiology and Sterilization

65. Examples of bacteria are
    (a) yeasts
    (b) viruses
    (c) bacilli
    (d) cocci

66. For growth, micro-organisms do not need
    (a) sunlight
    (b) moisture
    (c) carbohydrate and protein
    (d) suitable temperature

67. Under very adverse conditions what happens to most viruses?
    (a) they die
    (b) they cease to multiply
    (c) they form spores
    (d) they become quiescent

68. What are the main ways of killing micro-organisms on endodontic instruments after each patient?
    (a) flaming
    (b) immersion in antiseptics
    (c) dry heat sterilization
    (d) irradiation
    (e) glass bead sterilization

69. All spores can be killed by
    (a) chlorhexidine 20% solution in water
    (b) autoclave for 3 minutes at 134°C
    (c) boiling water for 1 hour
    (d) glutaraldehyde 2% for 10 minutes
    (e) dry heat for 1 hour at 160°C

70. A true sterilization cycle is
    (a) steam at 126°C for 18 minutes
    (b) hot air at 120°C for 2 hours
    (c) water at 100°C for 10 minutes

71. After removal from the sterilizer, dental forceps should be
    (a) placed in water to cool
    (b) stored in disinfectant
    (c) dried on a towel
    (d) stored in a sterile container
    (e) stored in a surgery drawer

72. Cross-infection means
    (a) passing pathogens
    (b) an unknown infection
    (c) a type of virus infection
    (d) infection which multiplies easily

73. The main problem in turning on water taps with the hands is
   (a) contamination
   (b) the handles become slippery
   (c) it takes too much time
   (d) none of these

74. The main objective in washing hands in the surgery is to
   (a) remove dirt
   (b) remove blood and saliva
   (c) sterilize the hands
   (d) remove surface contamination

75. The main objection to the use of bar soap for hand washing is because
   (a) it is slippery
   (b) it is expensive
   (c) frequent use damages the skin
   (d) bacteria can grow on it
   (e) none of these

76. Between patients the slow-speed handpiece should be
   (a) sterilized
   (b) dry wiped
   (c) wiped with antiseptic in spirit
   (d) oiled then excess wiped off

77. Impression trays returned from the laboratory should be
   (a) cleaned and sterilized
   (b) sterilized and stored
   (c) washed and stored
   (d) cleaned and stored

78. When treating a patient, rubber gloves are worn mainly to
   (a) protect the wearer
   (b) protect the patient
   (c) prevent needlestick injury
   (d) protect against saliva

79. Detergent cleaners should not be used in suction systems because they
   (a) are too powerful
   (b) are not antiseptic
   (c) can damage electric motors
   (d) do not remove blood

80. The best method of cleaning hands in the surgery is to
   (a) wash in chlorhexidine for 2 minutes, and dry on a paper towel
   (b) scrub with antiseptic soap for 3 minutes and dry on a paper towel
   (c) wash with antiseptic soap then with surgical spirit and dry in air
   (d) wash with hot water and dry in hot air
   (e) scrub with hot water and dry on a hand towel

81. After treatment of an inoculation-risk patient, work surfaces should be cleaned with
   (a) hydrogen peroxide 10%
   (b) methylated spirits
   (c) aldehyde 2% solution
   (d) chlorhexidine 2% in water
   (e) sodium hypochlorite 1000 p.p.m.

82. Which organisms are most likely to lead to which condition?
   (1) streptococci
   (2) *Salmonella*
   (3) *Treponema*
   (4) pneumococci
   (5) lactobacilli
   (6) *Candida*
   (7) staphylococci
   (8) viruses

   (a) denture sore mouth
   (b) sore throat
   (c) boils
   (d) acute ulcerative gingivitis
   (e) aphthous ulcers

Materials

83. For accuracy, both the alginate powder and the water for mixing should be at a temperature of
    (a) 37°C   (b) 37°F   (c) 70°F   (d) 98°F

84. Hydrocolloid impression materials are
    (a) irreversible   (c) inelastic
    (b) reversible   (d) brittle

85. If an alginate impression cannot be cast immediately it should be
    (a) stored in water
    (b) left to dry, then placed in a plastic bag
    (c) wrapped in a damp cloth, then placed in a polythene bag
    (d) placed in a refrigerator
    (e) wrapped in a dry tissue and placed in a box

86. After removal from the mouth, all alginate impressions should be washed to
    (a) remove saliva and food debris
    (b) sharpen detail on the impression
    (c) cool the impression
    (d) stop chemical reactions in the alginate
    (e) complete the setting

87. Which is correct? Plaster of Paris
    (a) originally came from the ground under Paris
    (b) models can be ground down for re-use
    (c) is never used in the mouth
    (d) has to be mixed with special plastic to make it harden

88. Pink wax sheets are normally used in dentistry for
    (a) wax forms for gold inlays
    (b) protecting models
    (c) locating denture over-extension
    (d) protecting new anterior restorations
    (e) occlusal registration

89. Glass ionomer cement contains
    (a) silica particles   (c) silicone material
    (b) phosphoric acid   (d) methyl methacrylate

90. The setting of glass ionomer cements is due to
    (a) moisture   (c) white light
    (b) chemical reaction   (d) body heat

91. After placement of glass ionomer cement the DA should have ready to cover the restoration
    (a) nothing   (d) eugenol
    (b) petroleum jelly   (e) fluoride solution
    (c) copal varnish

92. Plaster of Paris can be used to take impressions for
    (a) bridges
    (b) partial dentures
    (c) reline of full dentures
    (d) orthodontic appliances
    (e) new full dentures

93. Soft linings are used in dentistry
    (a) under porcelain crowns
    (b) in deep cavities
    (c) on the fitting surfaces of dentures
    (d) under composite fillings
    (e) in trays to store sharp instruments

94. Which materials are added to the periphery of special trays to produce a functional edge fit ?
    (a) composition
    (b) peripheral seal
    (c) gutta percha
    (d) alginate
    (e) sticky wax

95. Which materials are rarely used on their own for full denture reline impressions?
    (a) elastomers
    (b) zinc oxide-eugenol paste
    (c) composition
    (d) tissue conditioner
    (e) peripheral seal

96. The base of a full denture is usually made from
    (a) stainless steel
    (b) acrylic
    (c) PVC
    (d) gold
    (e) polycarbonate

97. Which materials are not used to make the teeth on dentures ?
    (a) plastic
    (b) porcelain
    (c) gold
    (d) composite
    (e) silicate

98. Articulating paper is used to
    (a) check the fit of a crown
    (b) check the fit of a denture
    (c) open the bite
    (d) locate premature occlusal contact
    (e) check the fit of contact points

99. A tissue conditioner is
    (a) a powder sprinkled on to the fitting surface of a denture
    (b) a powder-liquid cream applied to the fitting surface of a denture
    (c) a wax which is soft at mouth temperature
    (d) a constituent of alginate powder

100. Gutta percha is
    (a) a rubber material
    (b) a man-made plastic
    (c) used in mouth impressions
    (d) used as a soft lining
    (e) used as a temporary denture

Prosthetics

101. Prosthesis means
   (a) oral hygiene instructions
   (b) the application of topical fluoride
   (c) a type of general anaesthetic
   (d) an artificial replacement for lost tissue
   (e) calcification of teeth

102. Loose ill-fitting dentures can cause
   (a) ulceration of the mouth
   (b) excessive wear of the fitting surface
   (c) problems in making new dentures
   (d) the dentures to become coated with calculus
   (e) the tongue to grow larger

103. Gradual loosening of dentures is due to
   (a) being worn too often
   (b) not being worn full time
   (c) shrinkage of the plastic
   (d) changes in the alveolar bone
   (e) changes in the mucous membrane

104. Which of the following materials is suitable on its own for full denture final impressions?
   (a) alginate
   (b) composition sheets
   (c) composition sticks
   (d) plaster of Paris
   (e) gutta percha

105. When a plaster of Paris impression is removed from the mouth it may break. The pieces should be
   (a) thrown away
   (b) put aside for the dental surgeon to deal with
   (c) put in a bag and sent to the laboratory

106. An alginate impression mix should be well spatulated in order to
   (a) mix the powder with water
   (b) reduce air bubbles
   (c) slow down the setting time
   (d) include air
   (e) speed up setting time

107. To help prevent retching with alginate impressions the DA should make the mix
   (a) softer than usual
   (b) slightly warmer
   (c) hot
   (d) stiff

108. The reason for holes in impression trays is to
   (a) allow escape of excess impression material
   (b) reduce the weight of the tray
   (c) allow escape of air trapped in the impression material
   (d) allow the operator to see when the tray is finally seated
   (e) anchor the impression material.

109. A patient brings in a partial denture with a broken lingual bar. This can be accepted for repair without reference to a dentist.
(a) True
(b) False

110. Materials commonly used for the final impressions for partial dentures are
(a) plaster of Paris
(b) composition
(c) alginate
(d) elastomers
(e) zinc oxide-eugenol

111. The objective at the impression stage for full dentures is to
(a) reproduce the shape of the patient's jaws
(b) obtain a print of the denture-bearing area
(c) obtain a model of the soft tissues of the mouth
(d) obtain a model of the jaws

112. The main objective in taking an impression in a special tray is to
(a) obtain a better outline for the new denture
(b) cover the maximum gingival surface
(c) obtain an accurate impression of all denture-bearing tissues
(d) reduce the number of eases of the denture

113. During the construction of full dentures, the objective at the bite stage is to record the
(a) relationshp of the dental arches to the skull
(b) vertical space between the patient's jaws
(c) vertical and antero-posterior relationship of the jaws
(d) position of the teeth
(e) the patient's 'bite' in wax

114. The main use of the Willis bite gauge is to
(a) measure vertical height
(b) measure length of the teeth
(c) record the way the teeth meet
(d) mark centre line of the face

115. In the construction of full dentures, some of the objectives at the try-in stage are to check the
(a) number of teeth
(b) fit of the denture
(c) peripheral outline
(d) shade of the wax
(e) vertical dimension

116. The objective at the fit stage of full dentures is
(a) only to give the patient the dentures
(b) to check the fit and carry out any necessary grinding
(c) to ease sore spots
(d) only to fit the dentures and check the appearance

117. Patient instructions in the care of acrylic dentures should include
    (a) regular cleaning in a mild detergent
    (b) always wear them at night
    (c) regular cleaning with an abrasive cleaner
    (d) not to drink hot drinks
    (e) cleaning over a bowl of water

118. To help get used to new full dentures patients could
    (a) suck toffees   (c) wear one denture at a time
    (b) suck boiled sweets   (d) wear for short intervals only

119. When full dentures are worn the jaws
    (a) no longer shrink
    (b) shrink more rapidly
    (c) change more at the back of the mouth
    (d) change more at the front of the mouth
    (e) shrink fairly evenly and slowly

120. For most older patients full dentures should be replaced at least every
    (a) year   (c) 10 years
    (b) 3 years   (d) 25 years

121. The appearance of an edentulous patient can be improved if the dentures have
    (a) the correct position of the anterior teeth
    (b) the correct thickness of the acrylic flanges
    (c) the correct vertical dimensions
    (d) light-coloured teeth
    (e) small upper incisor teeth

122. The best way to clean acrylic partial dentures is to
    (a) clean them in the mouth   (c) wash under running water
    (b) soak them in bleach   (d) use toothbrush and
                                 toothpaste

123. Dentures should be cleaned
    (a) after each meal   (c) once a week
    (b) before going to bed   (d) twice a day

124. A patient brings in an acrylic full denture with the upper right labial flange missing. This can repaired without an impression.
    (a) True
    (b) False

125. A broken vulcanite denture should not be accepted for repair without reference to the dental surgeon because
    (a) it cannot be repaired
    (b) an impression is always required
    (c) only some types can be repaired
    (d) it is better repaired in the mouth
    (e) a new denture may be necessary

126. The selection of artificial teeth for replacement full dentures depends upon the
(a) patient's complexion
(b) size, shape and colour of the patient's natural teeth
(c) size of the patient's face
(d) time the patient has been without natural teeth
(e) space between the patient's dental arches

127. An articulator is
(a) a type of speech   (c) a trimmer for study models
(b) the way teeth meet   (d) a laboratory jaw framework

Radiography

128. To reduce dental radiation hazards to the patient
(a) the patient should wear a lead apron
(b) children should not be radiographed
(c) slow films should be used
(d) routine films should not be repeated within a year
(e) rapid developer should be used

129. To reduce hazards to herself the DA should
(a) never hold the film in the patient's mouth
(b) stand beside the patient
(c) correctly process films
(d) hold the film in the patient's mouth using artery forceps
(e) get the patient to operate the timing switch

130. Which films are not used intra-orally?
(a) periapical   (d) panoral
(b) interproximal   (e) bimolar
(c) occlusal

131. A shorter exposure time is required for films of lower incisor teeth than for upper molars because the
(a) teeth are smaller
(b) X-ray tube is further away
(c) film is closer to the X-ray tube
(d) angle of tube to tooth is greater

132. The light and dark parts on a radiograph are due to
(a) different absorption levels by the tissues
(b) extra radiation given off by the object
(c) varied exposure time
(d) the method of developing
(e) variations in emulsion thickness

133. A bite-wing radiograph will indicate to the dental surgeon
  (a) interproximal caries
  (b) calculus
  (c) interdental bone crest
  (d) the periapical condition
  (e) incisal caries

134. A periapical radiograph is taken to indicate to the dental surgeon
  (a) root morphology
  (b) non-vital teeth
  (c) interproximal caries
  (d) salivary calculus
  (e) enamel thickness

135. Bimolar or oblique lateral radiographs are taken to show
  (a) fractures and swellings of the jaws
  (b) the development of unerupted teeth
  (c) bone loss in periodontal disease
  (d) interproximal caries
  (e) a root in the antrum

136. An occlusal radiograph is taken primarily to show
  (a) the presence and position of unerupted teeth
  (b) submandibular salivary gland calculus
  (c) a root in the antrum
  (d) caries in the anterior teeth
  (e) the length of the incisor roots

137. A cassette and an intensifying screen are necessary for which films?
  (a) dental panoramic
  (b) bimolar
  (c) bite-wing
  (d) lower occlusal
  (e) periapical

138. Dental panoramic films are not usually taken to show
  (a) presence and position of unerupted teeth
  (b) early interproximal caries
  (c) bone loss in periodontal disease
  (d) periapical abnormalities

139. The reason a skeleton denture should be removed before taking bite-wing films is
  (a) danger of swallowing it
  (b) it may cause retching
  (c) radiation affects the denture
  (d) it absorbs radiation

140. Excess radiation may be reduced by
  (a) using fast films
  (b) using extra-oral films
  (c) increasing the distance between the X-ray cone and the patient
  (d) using a smaller aperture on the X-ray head

141. The X-ray machine should be switched off when not in use in order
  (a) to reduce radiation hazard
  (b) to prevent overheating
  (c) to save money
  (d) to stop wearing out

142. Which tissues are most likely to be damaged by radiation?
(a) hair and skin (d) nerves
(b) blood cells (e) bone
(c) reproductive organs

143. Which of the following is not an intra-oral film?
(a) bite-wing (d) panoramic
(b) periapical (e) occlusal
(c) bimolar

144. Infrequent taking of bite-wing X-ray films of children's teeth is probably attributable to
(a) lack of necessity (c) teeth are not calcified enough
(b) films are too large (d) under-prescribing by dentists

145. A safelight may be tested in the dark room by
(a) an exposure meter
(b) placing an open film beneath the lamp
(c) placing a coin on an open film beneath the lamp
(d) placing an open film in the dark room for two minutes
(e) none of these

146. Undue exposure of X-ray film to the dark room safelight leads to
(a) no change (c) fogging
(b) blurred image (d) mottling

147. What is the usual range of temperature for the developer?
(a) 168–175°F (c) 68–70°C
(b) 37–40°C (d) 68–75°F

148. Match the faulty radiograph condition in List I with the probable causes in List II.

List I

(a) yellowing of the radiograph
(b) herringbone pattern on radiograph
(c) mottling

List II

(1) developer too warm
(2) air bubbles in the tanks
(3) film in mouth the wrong way round
(4) film damaged by bending
(5) large temperature difference between the tanks
(6) insufficient rinsing after fixing

149. The reason for washing an X-ray film between developing and fixing stages is to
(a) aid chemical reaction (c) remove fingerprints
(b) remove unwanted chemicals (d) prevent overdevelopment

150. The reasons for 'fixing' a film are to
    (a) prevent streaking   (c) produce a matt finish
    (b) sharpen the image   (d) remove chemicals in the film

151. Match the faulty radiograph state in List I with the probable causes in List II.

List I

(a) very dark picture
(b) blurred picture
(c) partial image

List II

(1) too long in the developer
(2) developer not warm enough
(3) X-ray tube not properly lined up
(4) film moved
(5) overexposure to radiation
(6) insufficient rinsing
(7) film in contact with another in developing tank
(8) patient moved
(9) developer too warm

Anaesthesia and Extractions

152. Name the basic techniques of administering local anaesthetics
    (a) infiltration   (d) perineural
    (b) intravenous   (e) inhalation
    (c) intramuscular

153. Select from List I the most appropriate word to complete sentences in List II.

List I

(a) sensory   (d) peripheral
(b) motor   (e) anaesthesia
(c) central   (f) analgesia

List II

(1) painful sensations pass along .... nerves to the brain
(2) to move away from pain, the muscles receive impulses from the brain along ..... nerves
(3) interruption of painful impulses to the brain by means of chemicals is called .....

154. Dental surgeons are mainly concerned with pain sensations in which cranial nerves?
    (a) III   (b) V   (c) VI   (d) VIII   (e) X

155. Local anaesthesia can aid in the diagnosis of causes of pain.
    (a) True
    (b) False

156. An ideal local anaesthetic should have which of the following properties?
    (a) it works quickly
    (b) it wears off quickly
    (c) it can spread quickly
    (d) it irritates tissues
    (e) it can be sterilized

157. A slight colouring of the local anaesthetic solution
    (a) is normal
    (b) should be reported to the dental surgeon
    (c) indicates that the solution should be thrown away
    (d) occurs in stronger solutions
    (e) occurs if the solution is too warm

158. Precautions may be necessary when local anaesthetic solutions containing adrenaline are used if the patient is taking
    (a) analgesics
    (b) some antibiotics
    (c) antihistamines
    (d) certain anti-depressant drugs
    (e) cortico-steroid drugs

159. A surface anaesthetic is used in order to
    (a) give surface analgesia
    (b) control salivation
    (c) prevent bleeding
    (d) mark the injection site

160. Failure to obtain local anaesthesia may be due to
    (a) out-of-date solution
    (b) too much vasoconstrictor
    (c) weak anaesthetic
    (d) faulty technique
    (e) a blunt needle

161. Administering an infiltration local anaesthetic causes the tissues to swell.
    (a) True
    (b) False

162. The main reason why a disposable cartridge needle should not be resterilized is because
    (a) it may be blunt
    (b) it may break
    (c) the plastic would melt
    (d) the plastic sleeve cannot be resealed
    (e) sterility cannot be guaranteed

163. The strength of adrenaline in local anaesthetic solutions is
    (a) 1 in 100
    (b) 1 in 1000
    (c) 1 in 80
    (d) 1 in 80000
    (e) 1 in 10000

164. Give two reasons why vasoconstrictors are included in local anaesthetic solutions.
(a) to sterilize the solution
(b) to prolong the anaesthetic time
(c) to reduce haemorrhage
(d) to make the anaesthetic work faster
(e) to strengthen the anaesthetic

165. Partially used local anaesthetic cartridges can be used again.
(a) True
(b) False

166. Sedative drugs are a substitute for local analgesia.
(a) True
(b) False

167. Indicate which type of local anaesthetic technique is most likely to be used in each case
(a) regional   (b) infiltration   (c) topical

(1) extraction of both lower canines
(2) cavity preparation in lower molars
(3) deep scaling of upper molars
(4) removal of very loose root fragment
(5) extraction of abscessed lower premolar
(6) apicectomy of upper lateral incisor

168. Match the words in List I with the descriptions in List II.

List I

(a) intraneural   (d) general
(b) infiltration   (e) trigeminal
(c) topical   (f) regional nerve block

List II

An anaesthetic drug:
(1) applied to the surface of the skin or mucosa
(2) applied adjacent to a nerve trunk
(3) applied adjacent to the site of operation
(4) applied at some point along a nerve
(5) injected into a vein and carried to the brain

169. Local anaesthetic cartridges are not re-used because the
(a) rubber seal would leak   (c) risk of contamination
(b) glass may be cracked   (d) solution may be too weak

170. The nerves usually affected by a mandibular nerve block are
(a) anterior superior dental   (d) intra osseous
(b) long sphenopalatine   (e) inferior dental and lingual
(c) occlusal and buccal

171. Anaesthesia means loss of
(a) all sensation   (b) consciousness   (c) pain sensation

172. Analgesia means
(a) loss of all sensation   (c) loss of pain sensation
(b) state of unconsciousness   (d) a type of drug

173. Relative analgesia is
(a) comparing pain killers
(b) administering nitrous oxide plus air
(c) administering nitrous oxide with oxygen
(d) giving local anaesthesia with a 'dental gas'

174. Nitrous oxide is supplied in a cylinder coloured
(a) red   (d) blue
(b) black with white collar (e) grey
(c) orange

175. What is meant by cyanosis?
(a) blueness of skin usually associated with low oxygen
(b) a poisonous chemical in the blood
(c) discoloration of nitrous oxide gas
(d) excess CO_2
(e) a condition due to excessive alcohol intake

176. Which drug can be added to nitrous oxide/oxygen mixture to produce a smoother anaesthetic?
(a) halothane   (d) triplopen
(b) methohexitone   (e) methane
(c) haloperidol

177. The minimum percentage of oxygen normally given with nitrous oxide during a general anaesthetic is
(a) 5%   (b) 10%   (c) 0%   (d) 20%   (e) 25%

178. Premedication is
(a) thinking about a future event
(b) given to relieve after pain
(c) to help a patient recover from a general anaesthetic
(d) sterilization of the mucosa before giving an injection
(e) used to allay a patient's fears

179. The main disadvantage of oral premedication is
(a) a very high dosage is needed
(b) the effect is very variable
(c) the bitter taste
(d) the patient has to be starved
(e) patient's dislike of injections

180. Two hours after the injection of a sedation dose of diazepam most patients
   (a) would be asleep
   (b) would be fit to drive a car
   (c) could return home with an escort
   (d) could return to work

181. Extraction forceps are usually applied to the
   (a) crown of the tooth   (c) root of the tooth
   (b) alveolar bone   (d) gingiva

182. Straightforward extraction of a tooth involves breaking the
   (a) alveolus   (c) periodontal ligament
   (b) apical blood vessels   (d) periosteum

183. The surgical approach to an extraction is used because it is
   (a) more professional   (c) it is less painful
   (b) clinically necessary   (d) it is the best method

184. During removal of bone, surgical burs should be irrigated
   (a) to remove debris   (c) to keep them cool
   (b) to prevent blunting   (d) to stop bleeding

185. A dry socket is one without
   (a) blood   (c) saliva
   (b) bone   (d) cementum

186. Haemorrhage a few days after tooth extraction is probably attributable to
   (a) infection   (c) loss of vasoconstrictor effect
   (b) rinsing   (d) anaesthesia wearing off

187. Rinsing after a tooth extraction can lead to
   (a) bone infection   (c) increased blood flow
   (b) infected gums   (d) breakdown of the blood clot

188. Pericoronitis is inflammation
   (a) of the pulp   (c) around the crown of a tooth
   (b) around the brain   (d) of the periodontal ligament

189. Instruments to assist in the simple removal of roots are
   (a) rat-toothed forceps   (c) excavators
   (b) elevators   (d) broaches

Caries

190. Early smooth surface enamel decay shows clinically as
   (a) an opaque white patch   (c) a brown patch
   (b) chipping of the enamel   (d) a radio-opaque area

191. Caries occurs mainly in fissures and interproximal spaces because they are
(a) areas of weak dentine
(b) difficult areas for the dental surgeon to examine
(c) never in contact with saliva
(d) difficult areas to clean properly
(e) areas of weak enamel

192. Dental caries occurs in soft tissues
(a) True
(b) False

193. Dental caries always starts
(a) externally   (b) internally   (c) can be both

194. Dental caries does not occur in
(a) unerupted teeth   (d) the pulp
(b) partially erupted teeth   (e) supernumerary teeth
(c) fully erupted teeth

195. The carious process
(a) is bacteria converting carbohydrates to acids
(b) is acid foods attacking enamel
(c) is bacteria eroding enamel
(d) is plaque attacking the enamel
(e) involves proteolysis and decalcification

196. When caries has passed through enamel it spreads primarily
(a) along the amelo-dental junction
(b) into the pulp
(c) into the dentine
(d) into the cementum

197. Food is more likely to stagnate around teeth which are
(a) unopposed   (d) crowned
(b) unerupted   (e) spaced
(c) irregular

198. Research work has shown that the greatest incidence of dental caries is associated with
(a) sticky sugar as part of each meal
(b) sugary drinks as part of each meal
(c) sugar intake between meals

199. The commonest cause of a dental abscess in young people is
(a) gum disease   (c) erupting teeth
(b) injury   (d) pulp death

200. The pulp tries to protect itself against low-grade carious process
  (a) by increasing its blood supply
  (b) by forming reparative dentine
  (c) by forming an abscess
  (d) by producing painful sensations
  (e) none of these

201. Toothache is associated with
  (a) enamel decay   (d) exposed cementum
  (b) exposed interdental bone (e) early dentine decay
  (c) pulp exposure

202. Pulpal necrosis means
  (a) chronic inflammation of the pulp
  (b) a healthy pulp
  (c) partial removal of the pulp
  (d) total removal of the pulp
  (e) death of the pulp

203. Enamel caries differs from dentine caries because dentine
  (a) has a higher temperature   (d) has no nerve supply
  (b) is not bathed in saliva   (e) has a greater organic content
  (c) has a blood supply

204. Dental caries means loss of tooth substance due to
  (a) bacteria   (d) food and bacteria
  (b) chemicals in the mouth   (e) the enamel crumbling
  (c) sweets

Orthodontics and Children's Dentistry

205. Orthodontics is mainly concerned with
  (a) maladjustment   (c) mastication
  (b) malocclusion   (d) articulation

206. A removable orthodontic appliance usually needs to be adjusted by the orthodontist once
  (a) a week   (b) a month   (c) every three months

207. A supernumerary tooth means
  (a) an incisor tooth   (c) an unusually shaped tooth
  (b) an extra tooth   (d) a type of posterior tooth

208. The primary aim of orthodontics is to enable a patient to
  (a) have a reduced caries rate
  (b) clean teeth properly
  (c) talk properly
  (d) bite with teeth in any position
  (e) have well-aligned teeth

209. Crowding usually means that the patient has
    (a) too many teeth
    (b) canines which have erupted buccally
    (c) insufficient space for the third premolars
    (d) the correct number of teeth
    (e) larger teeth than the jaws can accommodate

210. A mother states that her child has two rows of lower front teeth. Is this condition
    (a) possible   (b) impossible

211. Removable orthodontic appliances should be taken out and cleaned
    (a) daily   (c) before going to bed
    (b) after each meal   (d) only by the dental surgeon

212. A patient with a damaged removable orthodontic appliance should
    (a) see the dental surgeon as soon possible
    (b) see the dental surgeon within a week
    (c) wait until the next appointment
    (d) continue to wear it if possible
    (e) leave it out immediately

213. A loose band on an orthodontic appliance should be pushed back into place by the patient, and left until the next appointment.
    (a) True   (b) False

214. Stainless steel bands of a fixed orthodontic appliance are held in place by
    (a) being a tight fit   (c) neither of these
    (b) cement   (d) both of these

215. Orthodontic brackets can be attached to teeth using
    (a) zinc cement   (c) epoxy resin
    (b) composite material (d) composition

216. Retained deciduous teeth and supernumerary teeth are possible causes of overcrowding.
    (a) True   (b) False

217. Deciduous teeth can cause malformation of the permanent teeth by
    (a) infection   (c) retention
    (b) pressure   (d) premature loss

218. Deciduous teeth are not sensitive to pain
    (a) True   (b) False

219. The proportion of the pulp to the crown of a deciduous tooth compared to its permanent successor is
    (a) greater   (b) about the same   (c) smaller

220. Deciduous teeth are not sensitive to pain from drilling
(a) True   (b) False

221. Endodontics can be carried out on deciduous teeth
(a) True   (b) False

222. Caries reaches the pulp of deciduous teeth quickly because
(a) there is no dentine   (c) the bacteria multiply quickly
(b) the pulp is larger   (d) the enamel is soft

223. Early loss of deciduous teeth can allow space for the premolars to close
(a) True   (b) False

224. Deciduous teeth are seldom filled with
(a) amalgam   (d) glass ionomer
(b) composite   (e) porcelain
(c) gold

225. A very broken-down deciduous molar tooth is usually restored by
(a) amalgam   (d) molar endodontics and
(b) post and gold crown   amalgam
(c) pulpotomy and glass   (e) pulpotomy and stainless steel
    ionomer   crown

226. A child has a temper tantrum in the surgery, the DA could
(a) slap the child's leg
(b) play a quiet supportive role to the operator
(c) take over from the operator
(d) fetch the child's parent
(e) none of these

227. Exposure of the pulp of an incisor tooth in a 7-year-old would be treated by
(a) pulpotomy   (c) neither
(b) pulpectomy   (d) either

228. Mouth guards are mainly worn to
(a) protect the lips   (c) prevent mouth breathing
(b) stop tongue biting   (d) reduce injuries to teeth

229. A blow to a permanent incisor tooth may result in the fracture of
(a) enamel   (d) alveolar bone
(b) dentine   (e) pulp
(c) the root

230. A permanent incisor which has been knocked out cleanly
(a) can never be replaced in its socket
(b) can usually be replaced in its socket
(c) has to be cemented in its socket
(d) has to be crowned before replacing in its socket

231. A dental surgeon would be more likely to carry out a pulpotomy on an incisor of a seven year old because
(a) the dentine is very sensitive
(b) there is not yet a nerve in the root of the tooth
(c) the cementum has not yet formed
(d) the pulp chamber is small
(e) the root apex is open

232. A young patient who has received a blow to a permanent central incisor tooth should be
(a) given an appointment within 24 hours, if possible
(b) told not to bother until the next regular appointment
(c) asked to make an appointment if pain persists after a week
(d) advised to attend the local hospital
(e) advised to see his/her medical practitioner

Conservation

233. Briault, sickle and pocket measuring are examples of
(a) paper points
(b) locking tweezers
(c) scalers
(d) probes
(e) spatulae

234. Tooth erosion is caused by
(a) excessive toothbrushing
(b) smoking
(c) excessive intake of fruit juice
(d) gastric regurgitation

235. A fissure is
(a) a carious line in a tooth
(b) a fracture in enamel
(c) a cleft lined by enamel
(d) a gap between filling and tooth
(e) the gap between adjacent teeth

236. The surface of enamel can be damaged by
(a) milk
(b) citrus fruits
(c) fizzy drinks
(d) alcohol

237. A root dressing is
(a) a temporary in a carious root
(b) medication in a root canal
(c) a periodontal pack
(d) a tooth socket pack

238. The term 'lateral condensation' is applied to
(a) plugging amalgam
(b) packing a root filling
(c) moisture at cavity margins
(d) dislodging forces on dentures

239. Amalgam is retained in a cavity due to
(a) the cavity shape
(b) the cavity lining
(c) bonding to the cavity wall
(d) enamel cement
(e) micro-leakage

240. Amalgam when inserted into a cavity is said to be 'plastic'. This means that it is
(a) soft and able to be handled
(b) made from acrylic or similar resins
(c) both
(d) neither

241. Immediately after insertion amalgam should be
(a) carved   (d) triturated
(b) burnished   (e) varnished
(c) polished

242. Amalgam is usually preferred to gold as a posterior filling material because of its
(a) strength   (c) better cavity retention
(b) appearance   (d) ease of use

243. The reasons for condensing amalgam fillings are to
(a) exclude moisture
(b) reduce the amount of mercury in the amalgam
(c) strengthen the amalgam
(d) minimize porosity
(e) bond the amalgam to the dentine

244. A dentine pin is used mainly
(a) to fix a crown to the root   (c) to remove dentine
(b) for precision attachments   (d) to retain amalgam fillings

245. If the electrical amalgamator breaks down, the DA could mix amalgam using
(a) a rubber finger-stall
(b) the palm of the hand and a finger
(c) an empty tablet bottle in which to shake it
(d) a mortar and pestle
(e) there is no alternative

246. Amalgam fillings are carved in order to
(a) reduce the weight of the filling
(b) aid mastication
(c) reduce breakage
(d) strengthen the filling
(e) speed the setting of the amalgam

247. Polishing of fillings
(a) reduces the chance of further decay
(b) makes the filling look nicer
(c) removes mercury
(d) strengthens the filling
(e) removes marginal ledges

248. Mixed amalgam should not be handled because
  (a) it makes the hands dirty
  (b) it may absorb moisture from the hands
  (c) mercury may be absorbed by the skin
  (d) it speeds the setting time
  (e) it slows the setting time

249. A radiograph of a traumatized permanent incisor tooth is taken to
  (a) check for a root fracture
  (b) see if the apex of the root is open or closed
  (c) see if the pulp is broken
  (d) check the vitality of the tooth
  (e) estimate the length of the root canal

250. Match the names in List I with the descriptions in List II.

List I

  (a) mummification   (e) devitalisation
  (b) pulpotomy   (f) necrosis
  (c) coronectomy   (g) polypus
  (d) pulpectomy

List II

  (1) complete removal of the pulp
  (2) partial removal of the pulp
  (3) death of the pulp
  (4) preservation of a dead pulp

251. Filing of a root canal is carried out to
  (a) make the canal round (c) clean the pulp chamber
  (b) clean the cementum   (d) clean and shape the root canal

252. Antiseptics are placed in the root canal mainly to
  (a) kill micro-organisms (c) bleach the tooth
  (b) stop pain   (d) arrest caries

253. Root canals can be safely irrigated with
  (a) household bleach   (c) sodium hypochlorite 1000 p.p.m.
  (b) normal saline   (d) sodium peroxide

254. A short root filling is likely to lead to
  (a) caries   (c) a chronic abscess
  (b) root fracture   (d) a periodontal abscess

255. A ruler is used during endodontic treatment to measure
  (a) the tooth   (c) the radiograph
  (b) root canal instruments (d) the width of the pulp

256. The use of a parachute chain is to prevent endodontic instruments
    (a) dropping on the floor   (c) being ingested or inhaled
    (b) getting lost   (d) getting loose in the sterile tray

257. Treatment to improve the appearance of the discoloured crown of an upper incisor tooth can include
    (a) bleaching
    (b) exposure to ultraviolet light
    (c) fitting a porcelain veneer
    (d) polishing with prophylaxis paste
    (e) conditioning the enamel

258. Detailed impressions of a jacket crown preparation are obtained using
    (a) irreversible colloids
    (b) elastomeric materials
    (c) zinc oxide paste
    (d) rubber impression materials
    (e) reversible hydrocolloids

259. Examples of impression materials elastic at room temperature are
    (a) silicones   (d) polyethers
    (b) composition   (e) zinc oxide-eugenol
    (c) alginate

260. In the past 'white' fillings were seldom used to fill cavities in posterior teeth because the materials available
    (a) reacted adversely with premolar and molar enamel
    (b) were difficult to use
    (c) wore away too easily
    (d) took too long to set
    (e) had poor colour matching

261. Gold crowns are fabricated in the laboratory by
    (a) machine pressing of warm metal
    (b) bending metal at room temperature by hand
    (c) casting molten metal into high temperature moulds
    (d) grinding out from a metal block

262. The core for a crown can be made from
    (a) dentine   (d) cermets
    (b) amalgam   (e) zinc oxide
    (c) composite   (f) glass ionomer

263. Porcelain jacket crowns are fabricated in a laboratory by
    (a) heating ceramic glass powder and water
    (b) casting porcelain at room temperature
    (c) pouring a soft porcelain dough into a mould
    (d) carving from a block of porcelain

264. A jacket crown can best be defined as an artificial replacement of
(a) tooth substance
(b) most visible tooth substance
(c) enamel and dentine
(d) enamel

265. Which materials are not used in the construction of permanent crowns for posterior teeth?
(a) porcelain   (d) acrylic
(b) gold   (e) aluminium
(c) silver

266. The shade of the labial face of a porcelain jacket crown is
(a) even all over   (c) lighter at the mesial side
(b) darker at the neck   (d) darker at the centre

267. Which materials are commonly used to construct temporary anterior crowns?
(a) acrylic   (d) zinc phosphate
(b) composition   (e) composites
(c) epimines

268. Which of the following does not indicate a type of crown?
(a) post   (d) basket
(b) veneer   (e) bevel
(c) jacket   (f) three-quarter

269. Crowns cannot be made on root filled teeth.
(a) True   (b) False

270. The main reason for the construction of gold crowns on molar teeth is
(a) to protect the enamel   (c) to replace a lost tooth
(b) for appearance   (d) to replace large loss of dentine

271. Porelain jacket crowns are seldom fitted for patients under 14 years of age because
(a) there is a risk of fracture
(b) the root will grow
(c) the clinical crown will alter
(d) the shade of the adjacent teeth will alter

272. The post for a post crown may be
(a) cast in the laboratory   (d) made using amalgam
(b) precast with a thread   (e) made from a paper clip
(c) precast smooth-sided

273. Materials used to construct a temporary posterior crown include
  (a) stainless steel crown form   (f) mouth-curing acrylic
  (b) copper ring   (g) amalgam
  (c) celluloid crown form   (h) gutta percha
  (d) zinc oxide-eugenol   (i) aluminium crown form
  (e) zinc phosphate

274. The crown preparations on the teeth supporting a bridge should
  (a) be parallel to each other   (c) converge
  (b) be parallel mesio-distally   (d) diverge

275. Which of the items listed should be laid out ready for impression of a root canal for a post and core to be made in the laboratory?
  (a) paper clip   (e) zinc phosphate cement
  (b) retraction cord   (f) elastomeric impression
  (c) plastic burnout post   material
  (d) impression syringe   (g) pink wax
                                   (h) plaster of Paris

276. Detailed impressions for a bridge are usually obtained using
  (a) alginate   (d) plaster of Paris
  (b) elastomers   (e) reversible hydrocolloid
  (c) zinc oxide paste

277. Which term is not normally applied to dental bridges?
  (a) suspension   (d) fixed-free
  (b) cantilever   (e) adhesive
  (c) fixed-fixed

278. Select the materials used for permanent bridges
  (a) gold   (d) porcelain
  (b) composite   (e) stainless steel
  (c) chrome-cobalt

279. Which of the following are important parts of a bridge?
  (a) arch bar   (d) pontic
  (b) abutment   (e) occlusal rest
  (c) crib   (f) clasp

280. A bridge is fixed to supporting teeth by means of crowns because
  (a) there is no other means of supporting a bridge
  (b) it is easier to construct in the laboratory
  (c) the bridge is less inclined to rotate
  (d) there is good resistance to secondary caries

281. The luting cement for fixing a bridge should
  (a) drop from the spatula
  (b) just fail to drop from the spatula
  (c) be of a thick creamy consistency
  (d) be stiff
  (e) be very runny

282. An adhesive bridge is held in place by
  (a) the roughened metal surface
  (b) dental cement
  (c) microfine composite
  (d) glass ionomer cement
  (e) clasps and cement

283. A 'high' dental restoration will
  (a) increase biting efficiency
  (b) increase 'he chances of fracture of the restoration
  (c) make the tooth tender
  (d) allow for wear of the restoration
  (e) not matter

Multiple choice

Answers

General

1. (d)	2. (a)	3. (a)	4. (d)
5. (c)	6. (a)	7. (e)	8. (e)
9. (e)	10. (b) (e)	11. (d)	12. (a) (d)
13. (c)	14. (b)	15. (d)	16. (d) (b)
17. (a)	18. (d)	19. (d)	20. (b)
21. (c)	22. (c)	23. (e) (d)	24. (c)
25. (c) (d)	26. (d)	27. (d)	28. (c)
29. (b)			

Oral anatomy

30. (c)	31. (b)	32. (c)	33. (c)
34. (a)	35. (e)	36. (a)	37. (c)
38. (c)	39. (e)	40. (d)	41. (e)

42. (l) (d)   (2) (h)   (3) (g)   (4) (b)   (5) (e)
43. (l) (h)   (2) (j)   (3) (c)   (4) (f)   (5) (d)

44. (b)	45. (l) (i) (2) (c) (3) (a) (d) (4) (b) (e) (f) (h) (j)

46. (c)	47. (c)	48. (d)	49. (b) (d)
50. (b)	51. (e)	52. (b)	53. (a)
54. (c)	55. (b)	56. (a)	57. (a)
58. (d)	59. (e)	60. (e)	61. (b)
62. (c)	63. (e)	64. (d)	

Microbiology and sterilization

65. (c) (d)	66. (a)	67. (a) (d)	68. (c)
69. (b) (e)	70. (a)	71. (d)	72. (a)
73. (a)	74. (d)	75. (c)	76. (a)
77. (a)	78. (a)	79. (c)	80. (a)
81. (c) (e)	82. (a) (6) (b) (1) (c) (7) (d) (3) (e) (8)		

Materials

83. (c)	84. (a) (b)	85. (c)	86. (a)
87. (a)	88. (e)	89. (a)	90. (b)
91. (b) (c)	92. (e)	93. (c)	94. (a) (b)
95. (c) (e)	96. (b)	97. (c) (d) (e)	98. (d)
99. (b)	100. (a)		

Prosthetics

101. (d)	102. (a)	103. (d)	104. (a) (d)
105. (b)	106. (a) (b)	107. (b)	108. (e)
109. (b)	110. (c) (d)	111. (b)	112. (c)
113. (c)	114. (a)	115. (c) (e)	116. (b)
117. (a) (e)	118. (b)	119. (e)	120. (c)
121. (a) (b) (c)	122. (d)	123. (a)	124. (b)
125. (e)	126. (a) (c) (e)	127. (d)	

Radiography

128. (a) (d)	129. (a) (c)	130. (d) (e)	131. (c)
132. (a)	133. (a) (b) (c)	134. (a)	135. (a) (b)
136. (a)	137. (a) (b)	138. (b)	139. (d)
140. (a) (d)	141. (a)	142. (a) (b) (c)	143. (c) (d)
144. (d)	145. (c)	146. (c)	147. (d)
148. (a) (6) (b) (3) (c)(5)		149. (b)	150. (d)
151. (a) (1) (5) (9) (b) (4) (8) (c) (3) (4) (7)			

Anaesthesia and extractions

152. (a) (d)	153. (1) (a) (2) (b) (3) (f)	154. (b)	
155. (a)	156. (a) (e)	157. (b) (c)	158. (d)
159. (a)	160. (a) (d)	161. (a)	162. (e)
163. (d)	164. (b) (c)	165. (b)	166. (b)
167. (1) (b) (2) (a) (3) (c) (b) (4) (a) (5) (b) (a)			
168. (1) (c) (2) (f) (3) (b) (4) (b) (f) (5) (f)			
169. (c)	170. (e)	171. (a)	172. (c)
173. (c)	174. (d)	175. (a)	176. (a)
177. (d)	178. (e)	179. (b)	180. (c)
181. (c)	182. (b) (c)	183. (b)	184. (a) (c)
185. (a)	186. (a)	187. (c)	188. (c)
189. (b)			

Caries

190. (a)	191. (d)	192. (b)	193. (a)
194. (a)	195. (e)	196. (c)	197. (a) (c)
198. (c)	199. (d)	200. (b)	201. (c) (e)
202. (e)	203. (e)	204. (d)	

Orthodontics and children's dentistry

205. (b)	206. (b)	207. (b)	208. (e)
209. (d) (e)	210. (a)	211. (b)	212. (a) (d)
213. (b)	214. (d)	215. (b)	216. (a)
217. (a)	218. (b)	219. (a)	220. (b)
221. (a)	222. (b)	223. (a)	224. (c) (e)
225. (d) (e)	226. (b)	227. (a)	228. (d)
229. (a) (b) (c)	230. (b)	231. (e)	232. (a)

Conservation

233. (d)   234. (c) (d)   235. (c)   236. (b) (c)
237. (b)   238. (b)   239. (a)   240. (a)
241. (a) (b)   242. (d)   243. (b) (c) (d)   244. (d)
245. (a) (d)   246. (b) (c)   247. (e)   248. (c)
249. (a) (b) (e) 250. (l) (d)   (2) (b)   (3) (f)   (4) (a)
251. (d)   252. (a)   253. (c)   254. (c)
255. (b)   256. (c)   257. (a) (c)   258. (b) (d) (e)
259. (a) (c) (d) 260. (c)   261. (c)   262. (b) (c) (d) (
263. (a)   264. (b) (d)   265. (c)   266. (b)
267. (a) (c)   268. (e)   269. (b)   270. (d)
271. (a) (c)   272. (a) (b) (c)   273. (d) (e) (f) (i) 274. (a)
275. (a) (c) (d) (f) (g)   276. (b) (e)   277. (a)
278. (a)   279. (b) (d)   280. (d)   281. (b)
282. (c)   283. (b) (c)